Colombia

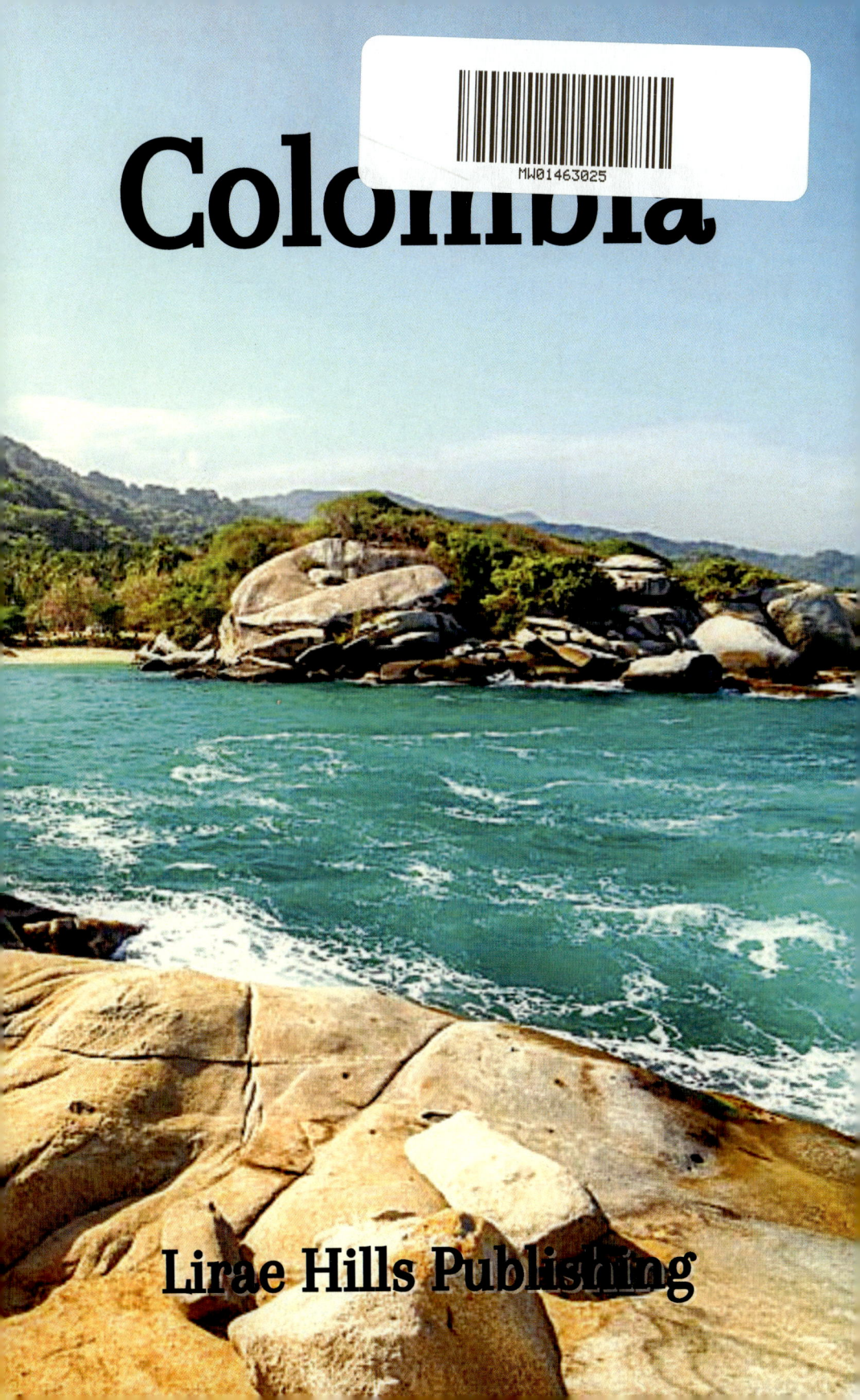

Lirae Hills Publishing

Copyright © Lirae Hills Publishing . All Rights Reserved. No part of this book may be reproduced in any form without the prior written permission of the author.

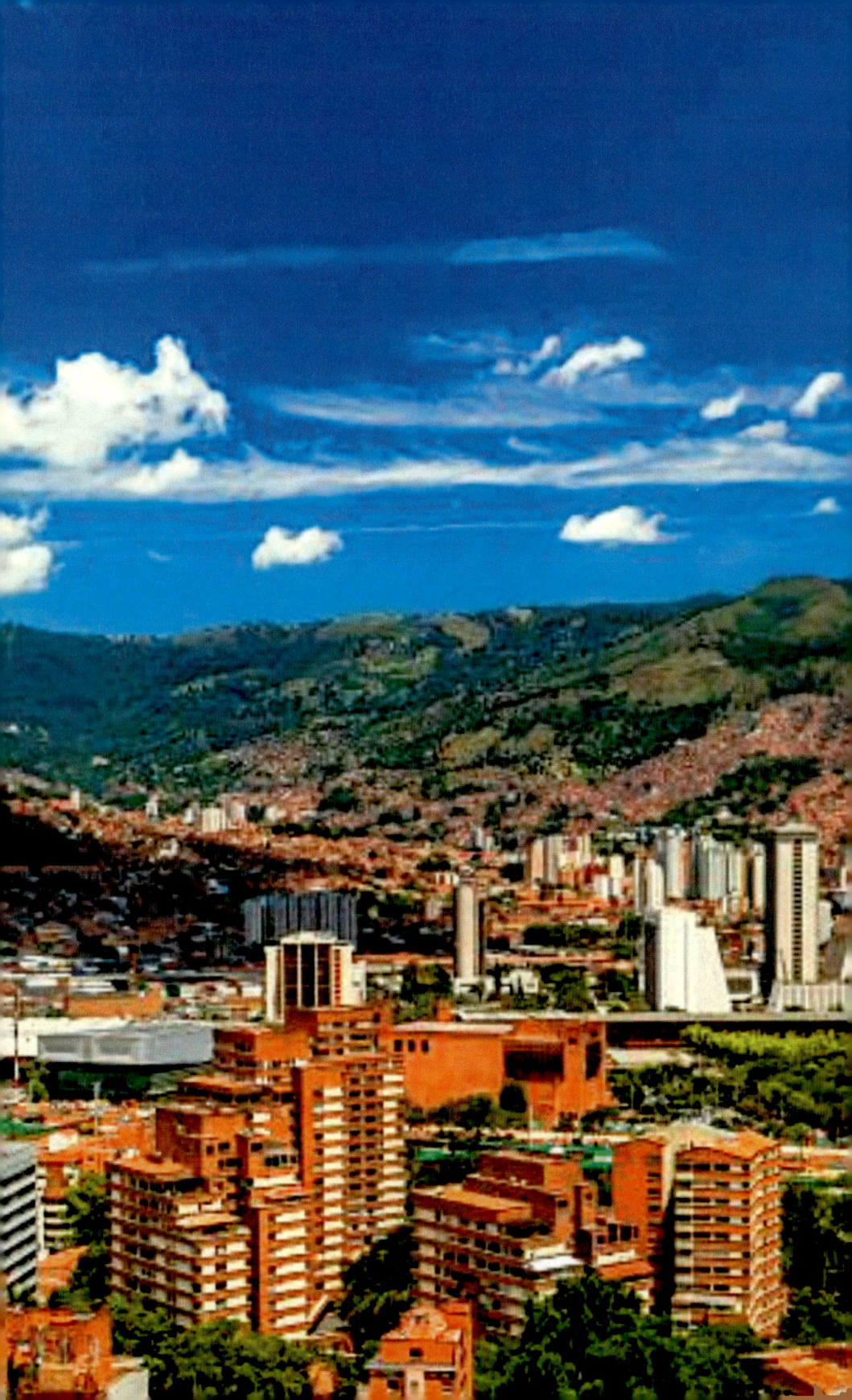

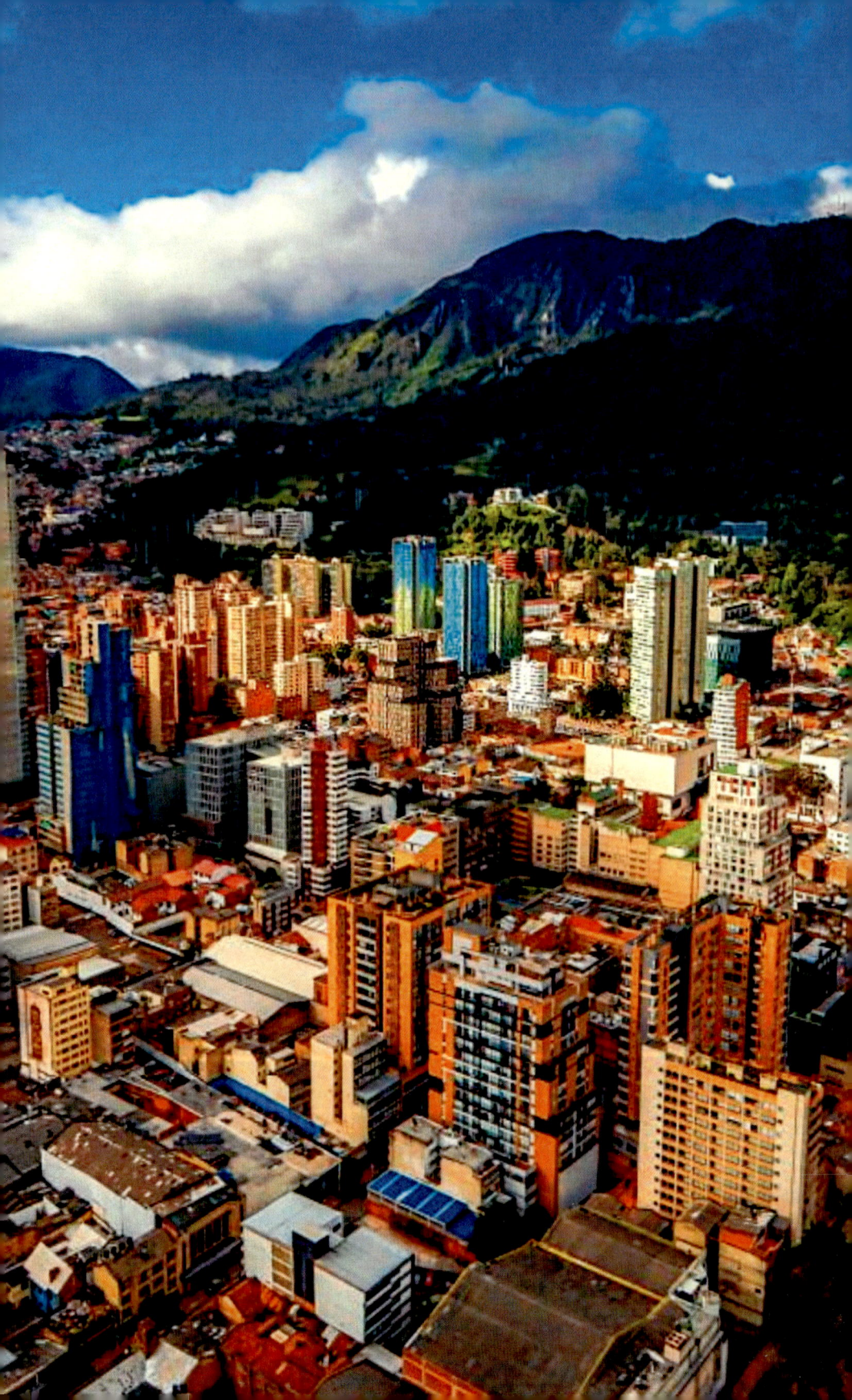

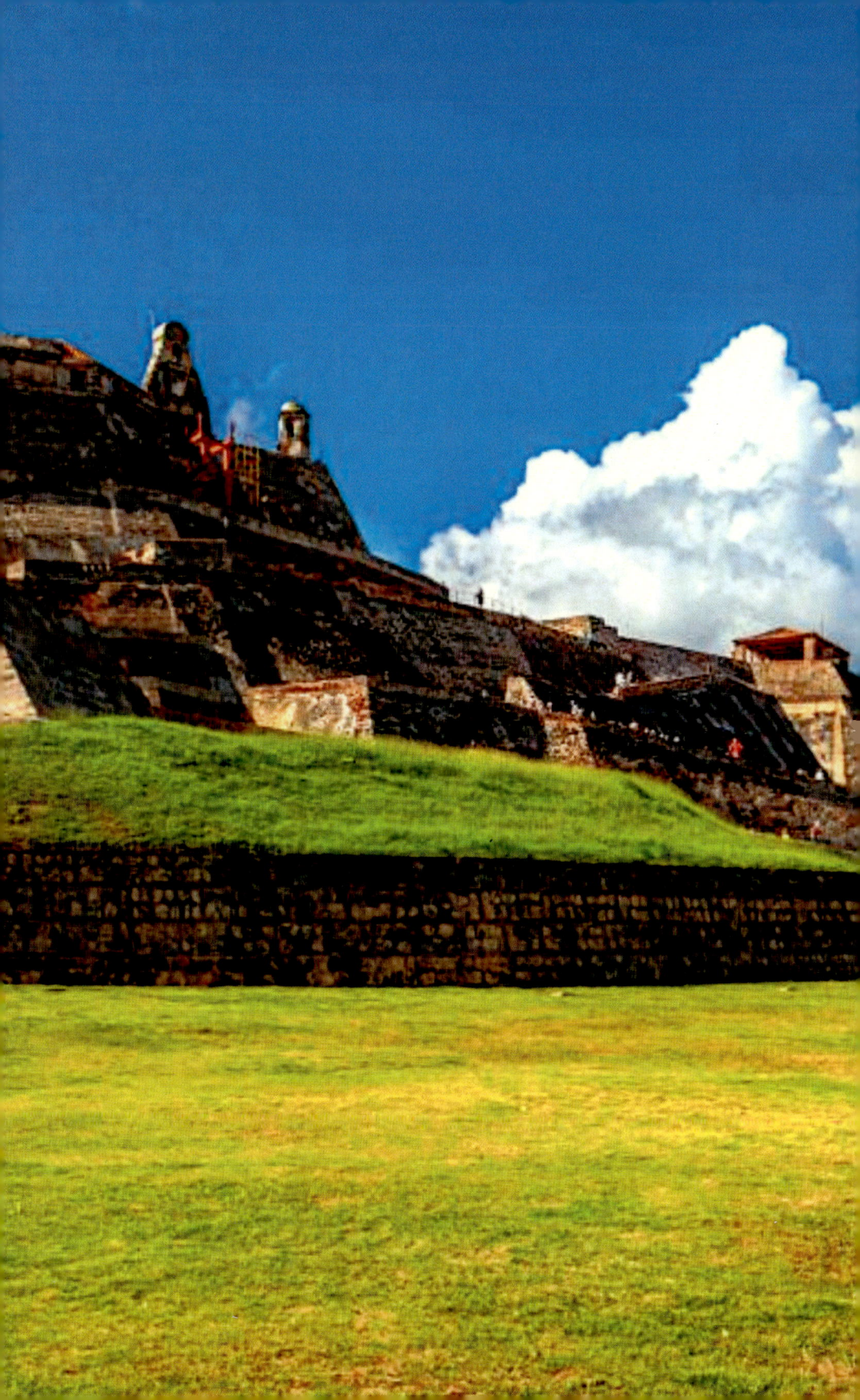

Cathedral of Cartagena

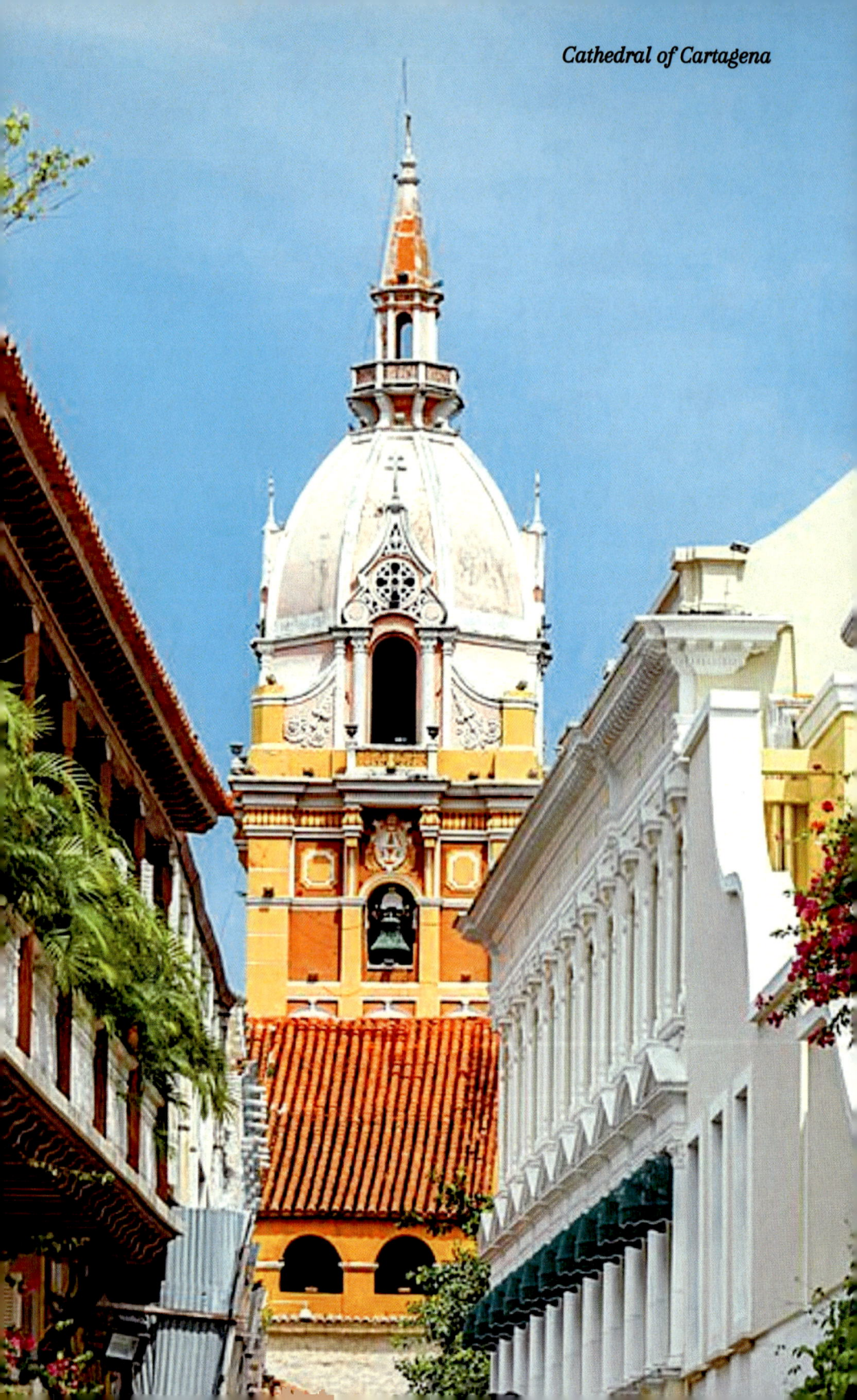

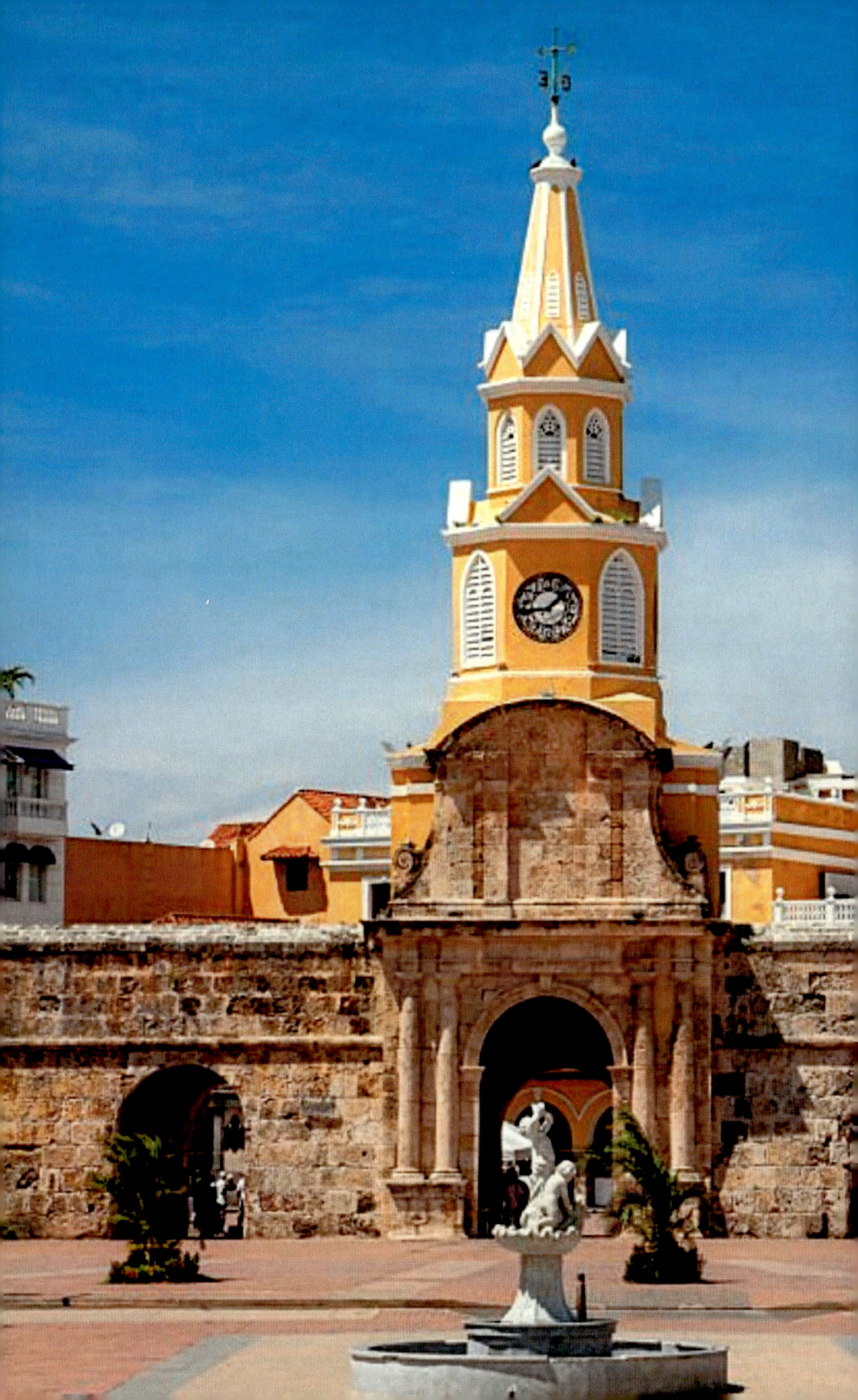

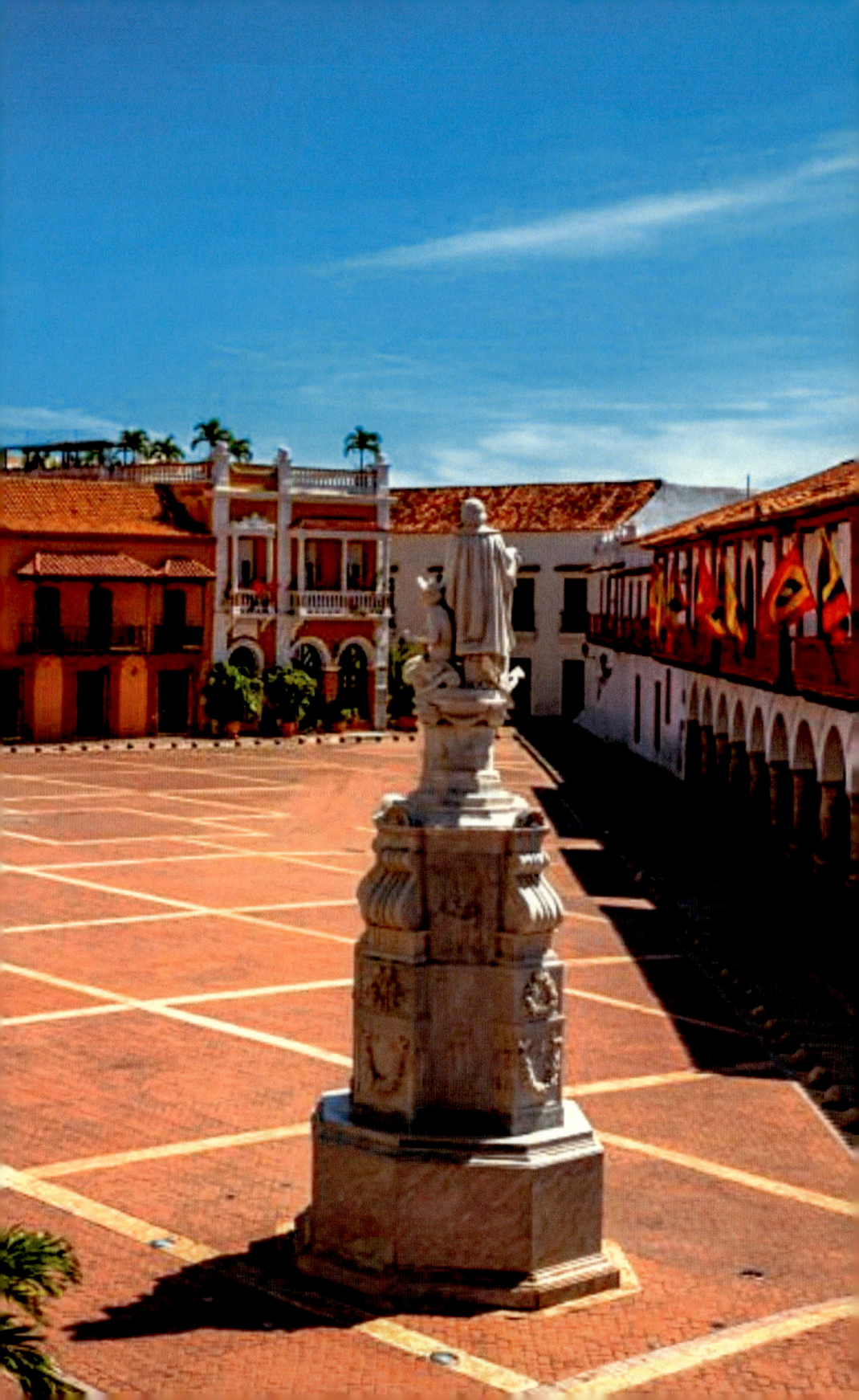

Tayrona National Park

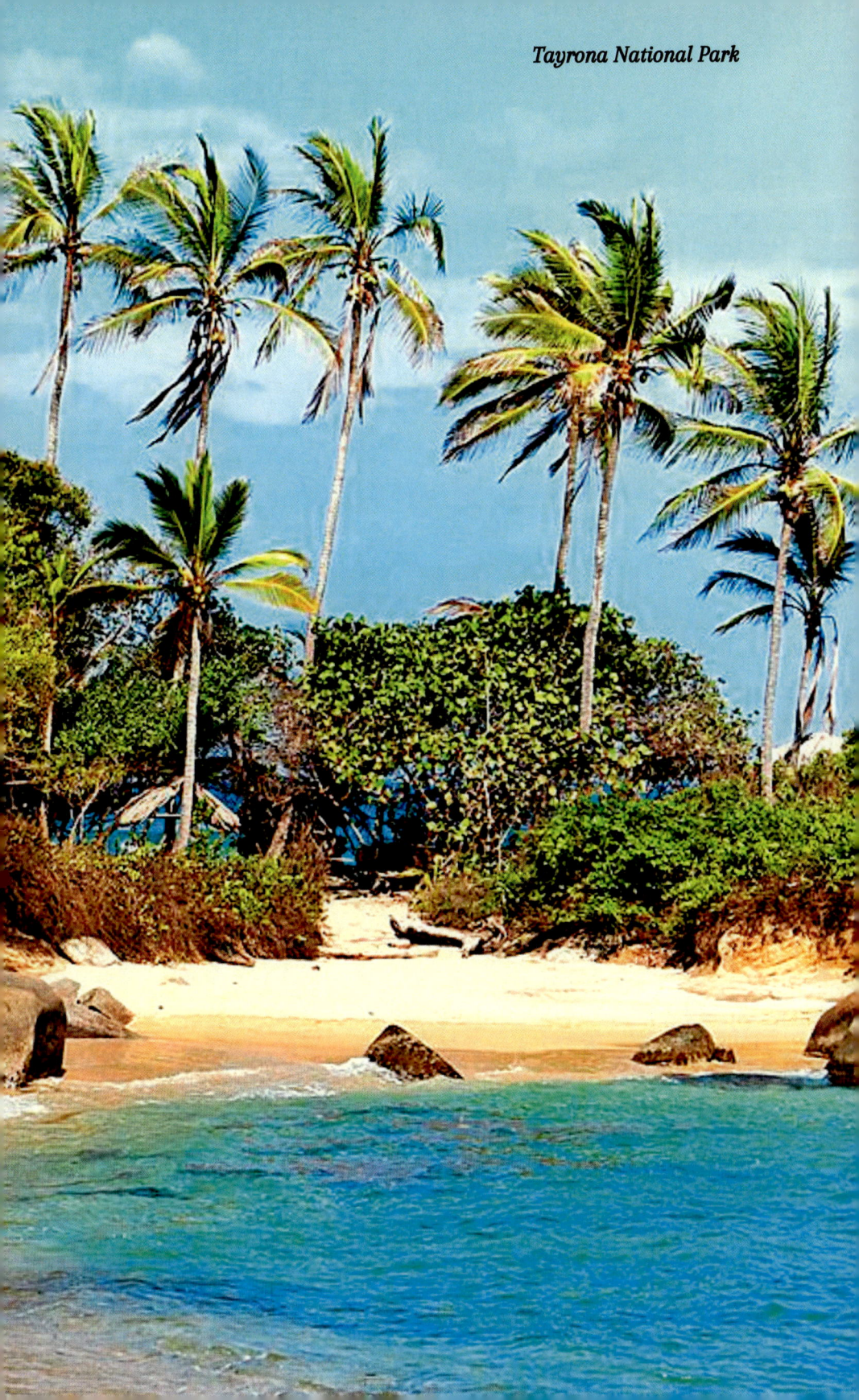

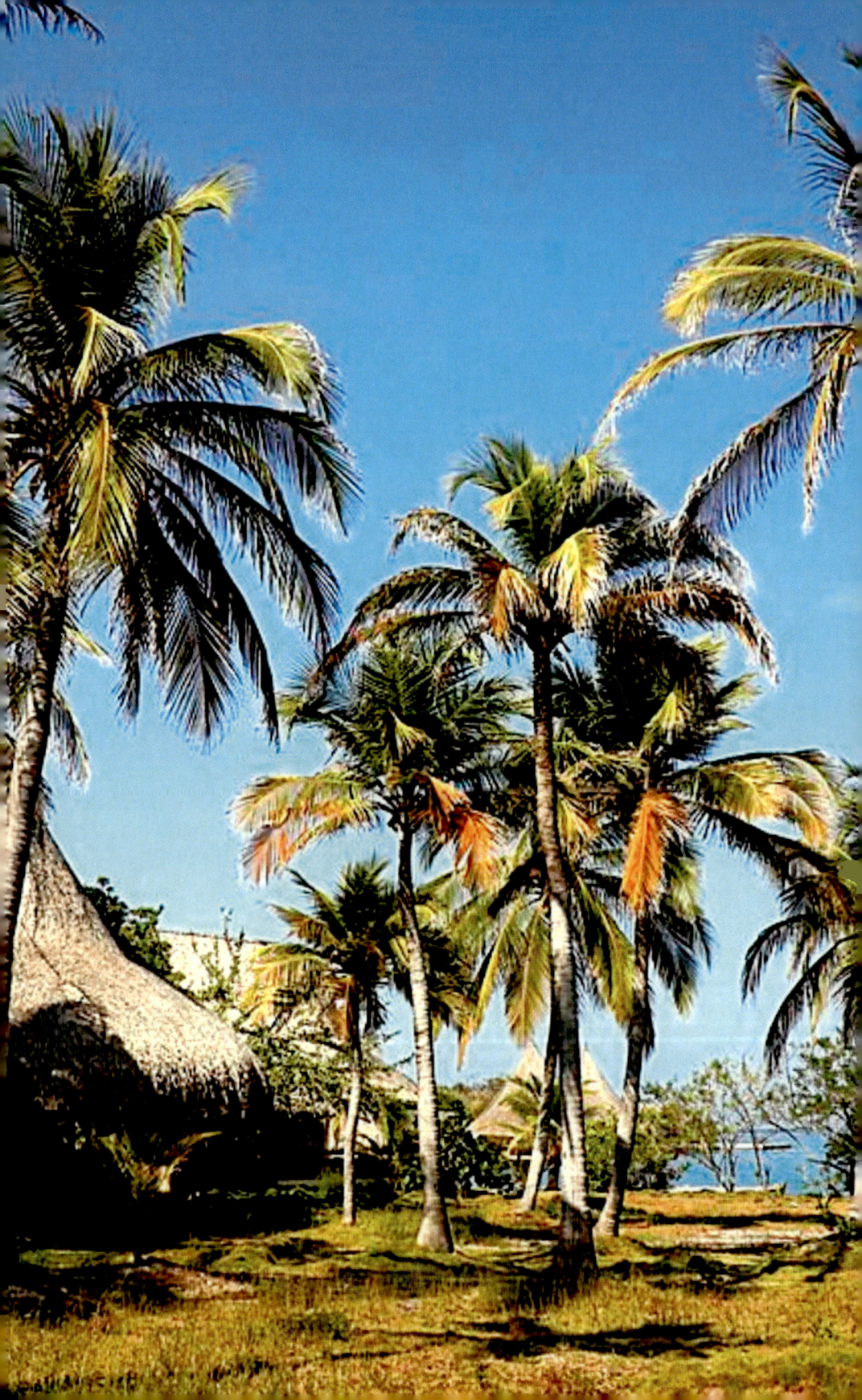

Morgan's Head

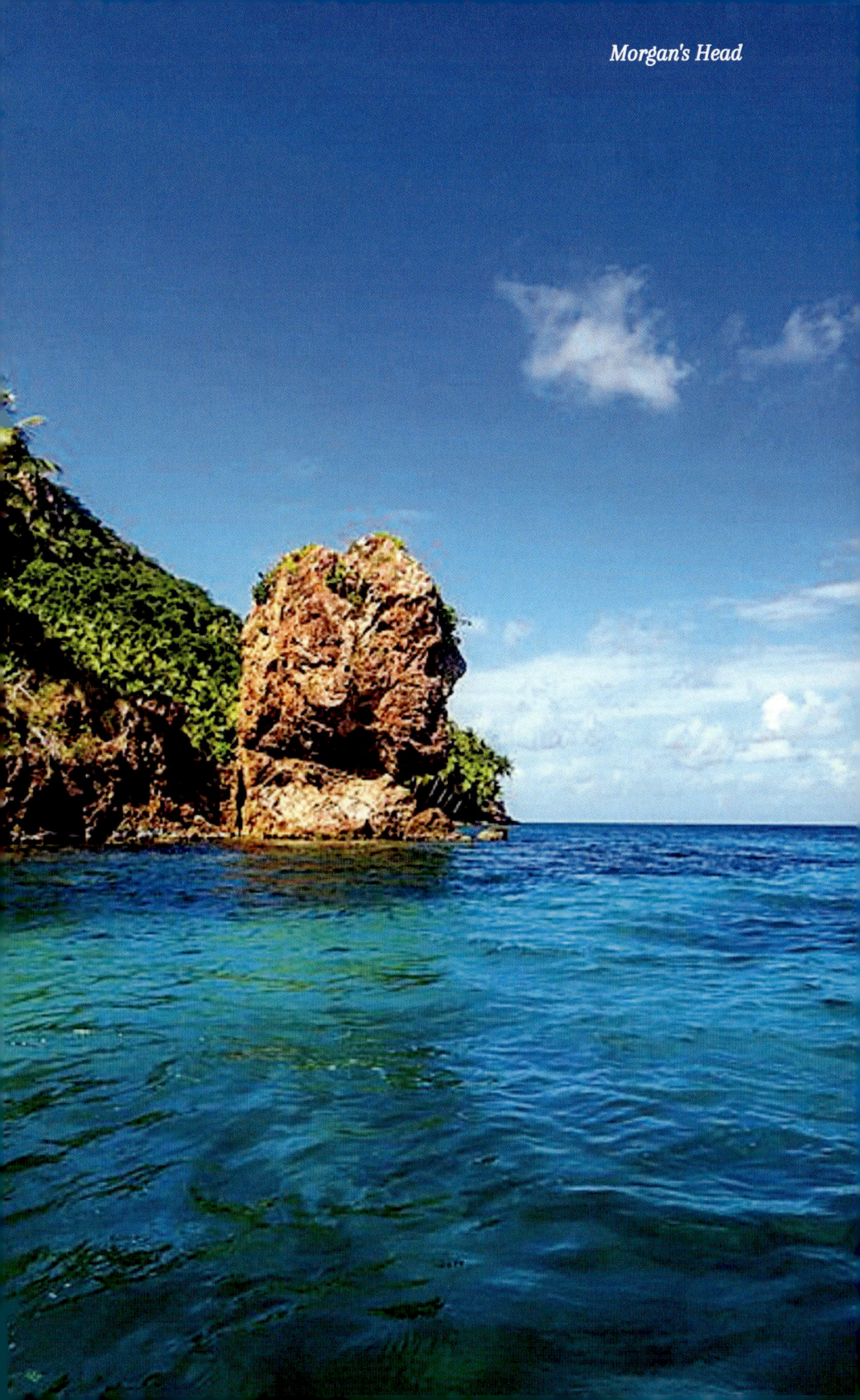

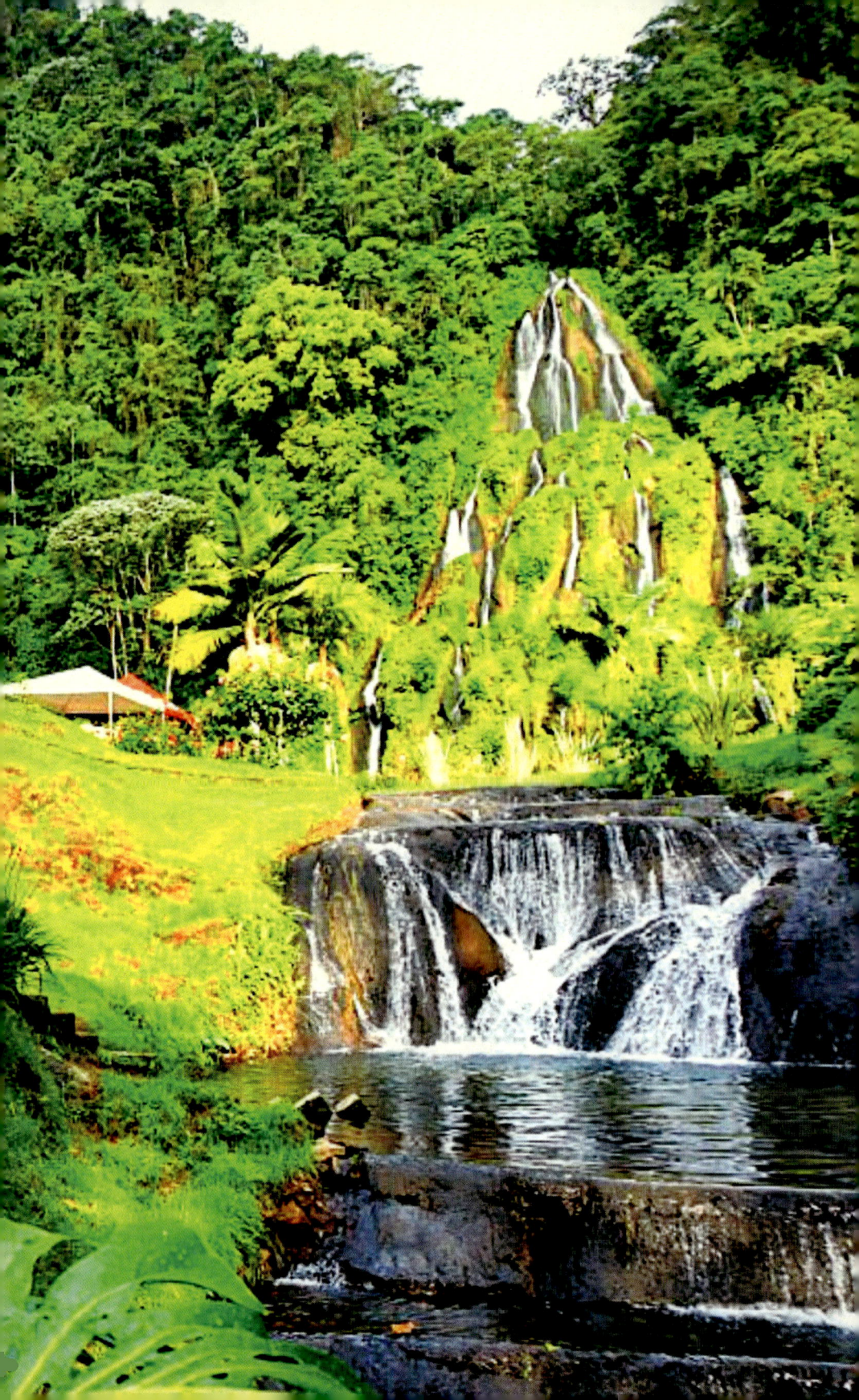

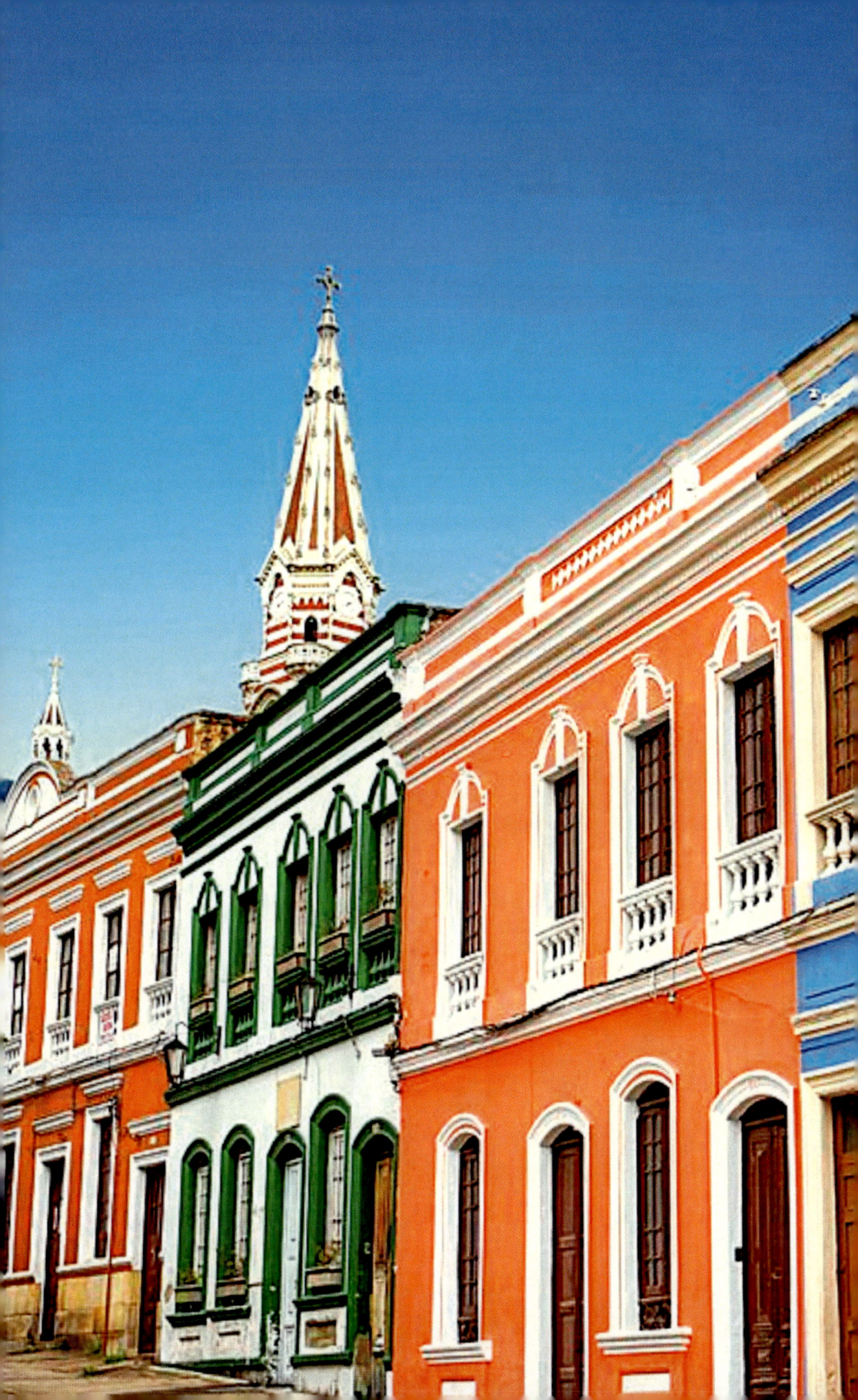

Monserrate Church

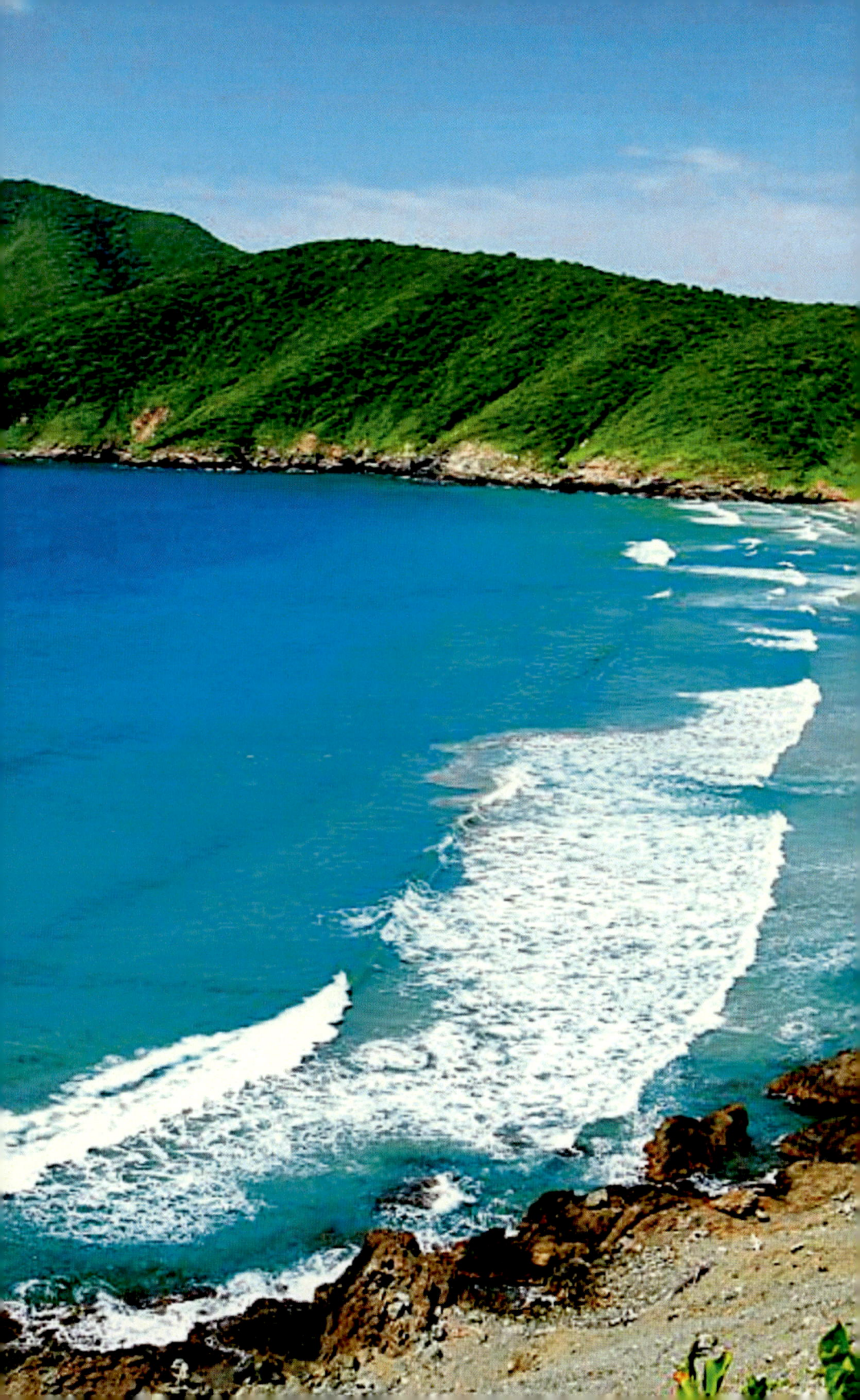

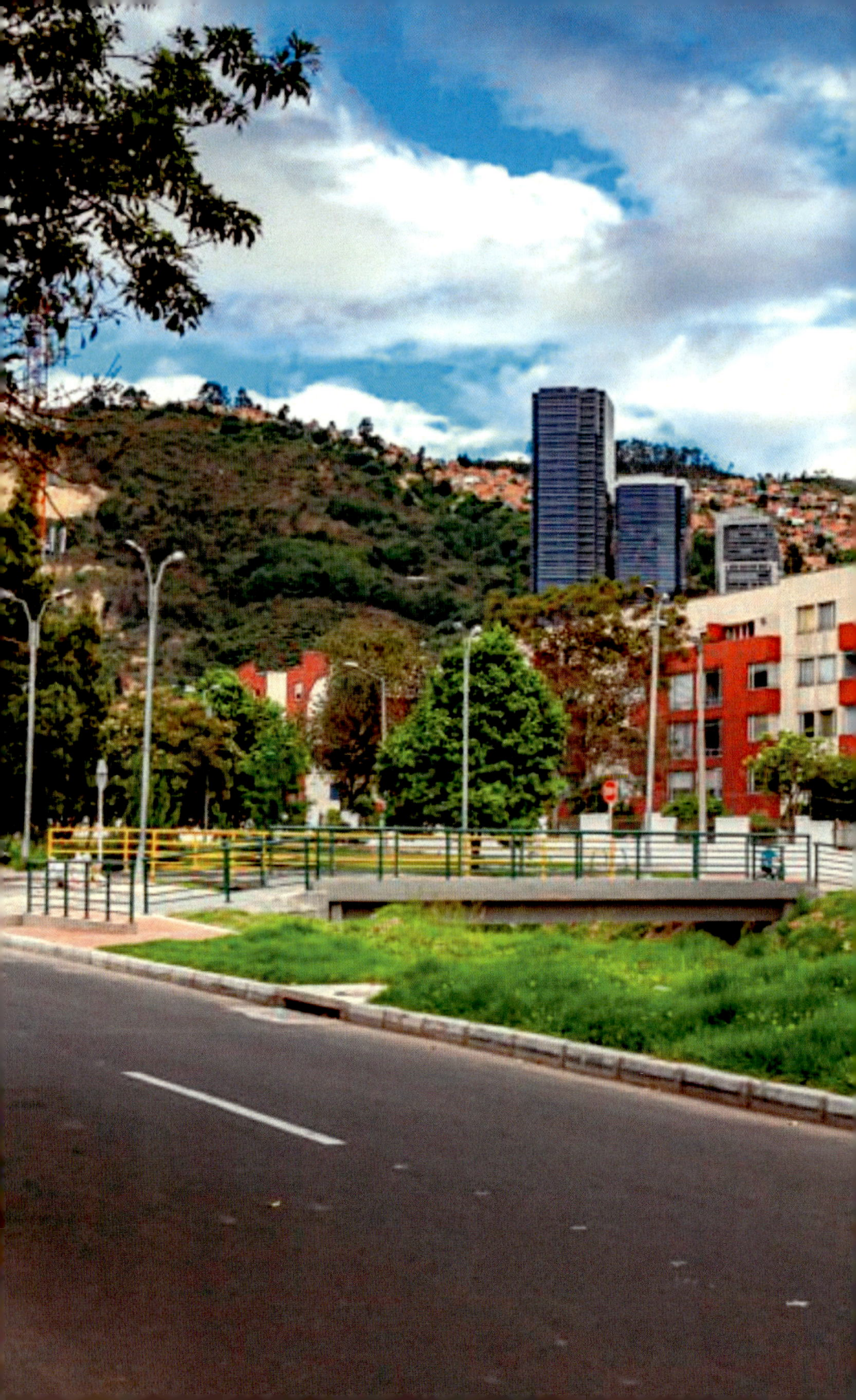

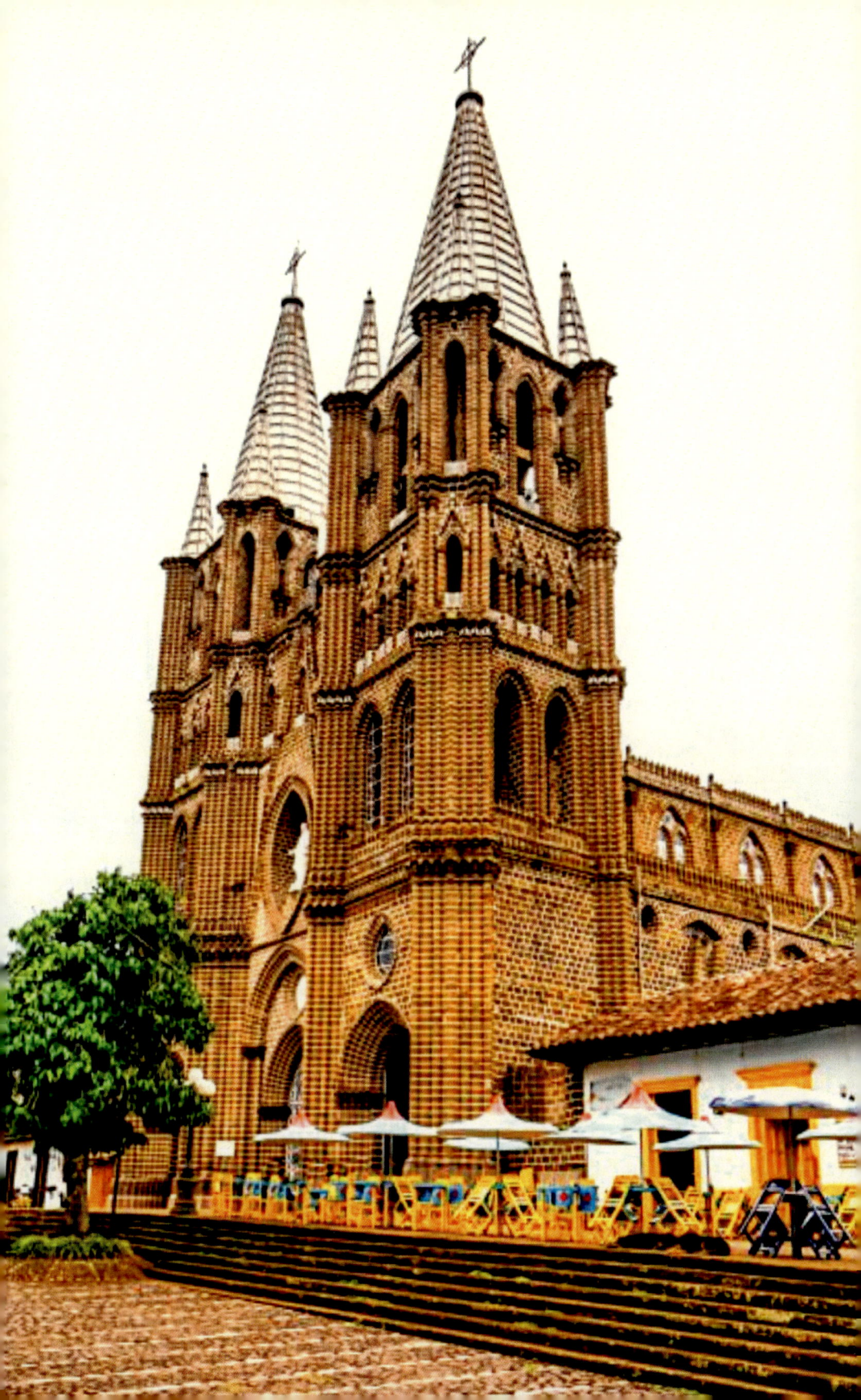

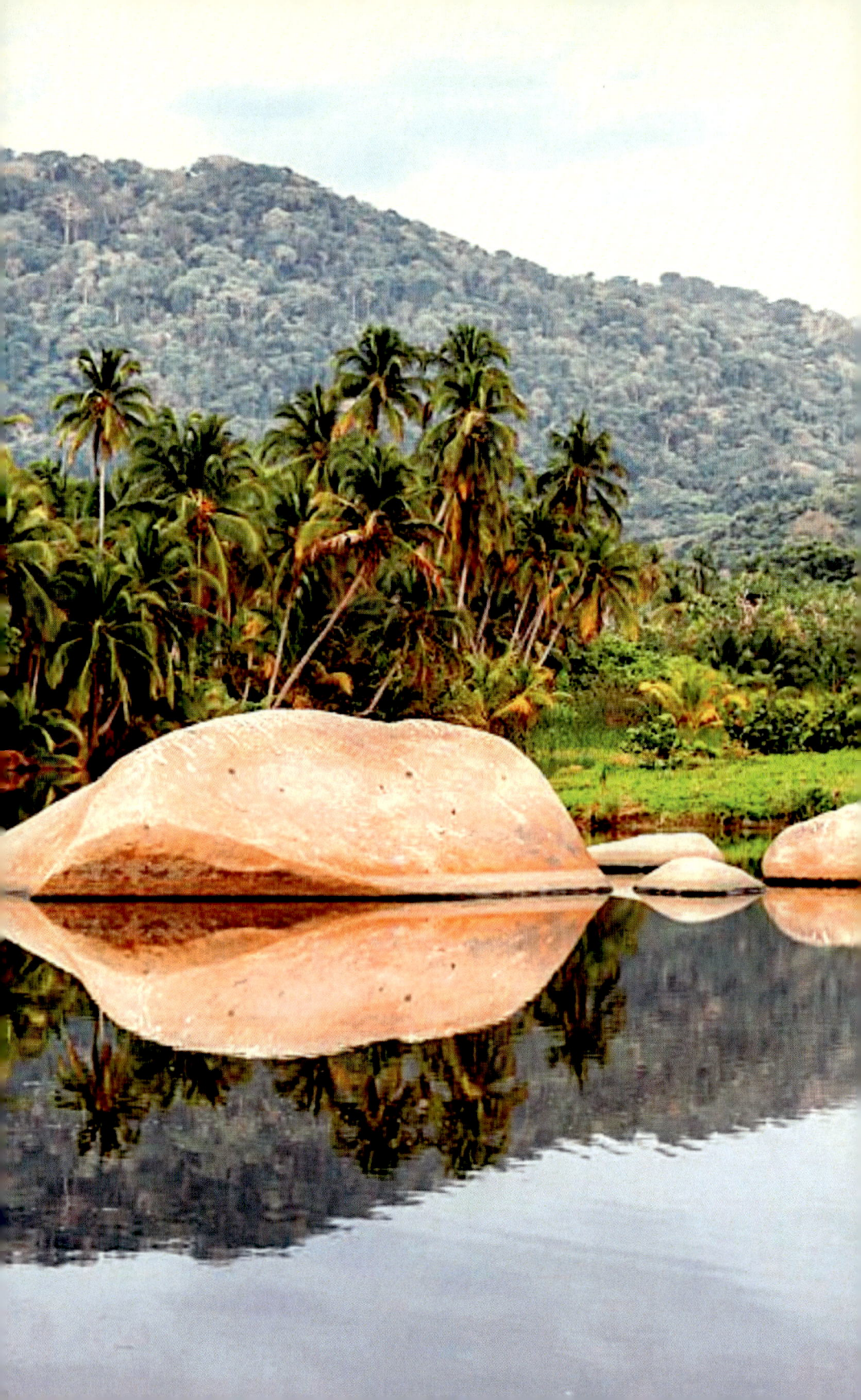

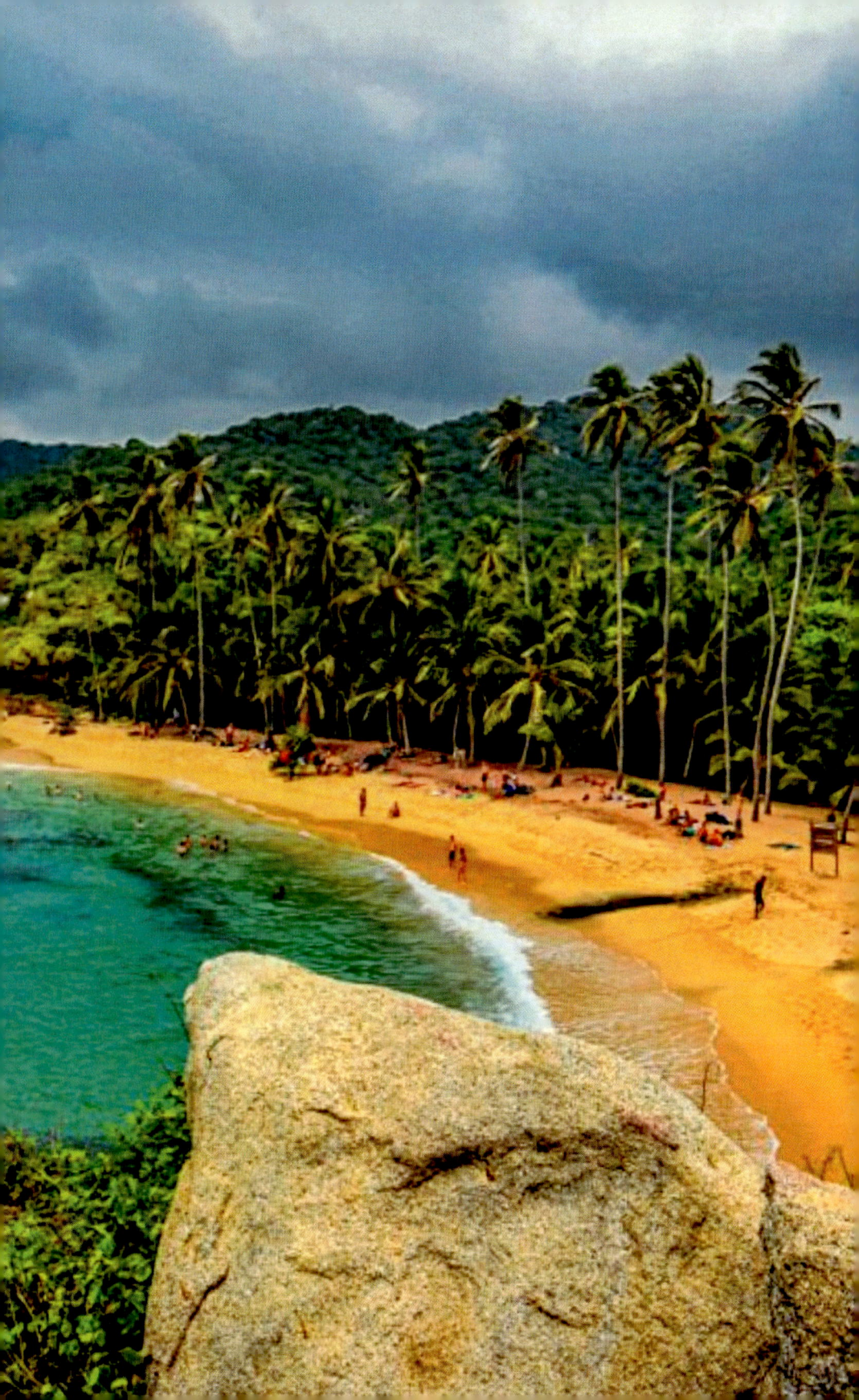

Cano Cristales

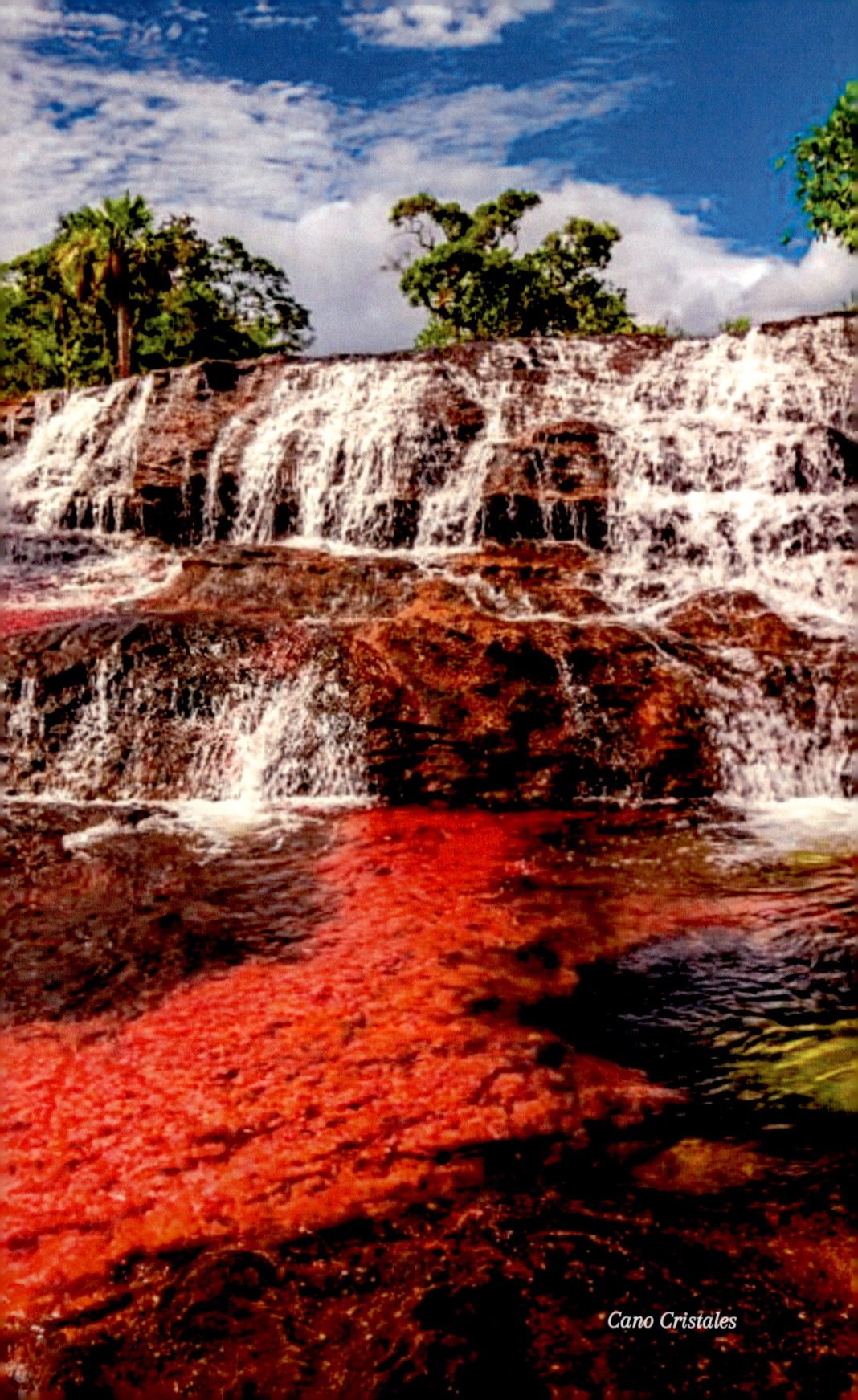

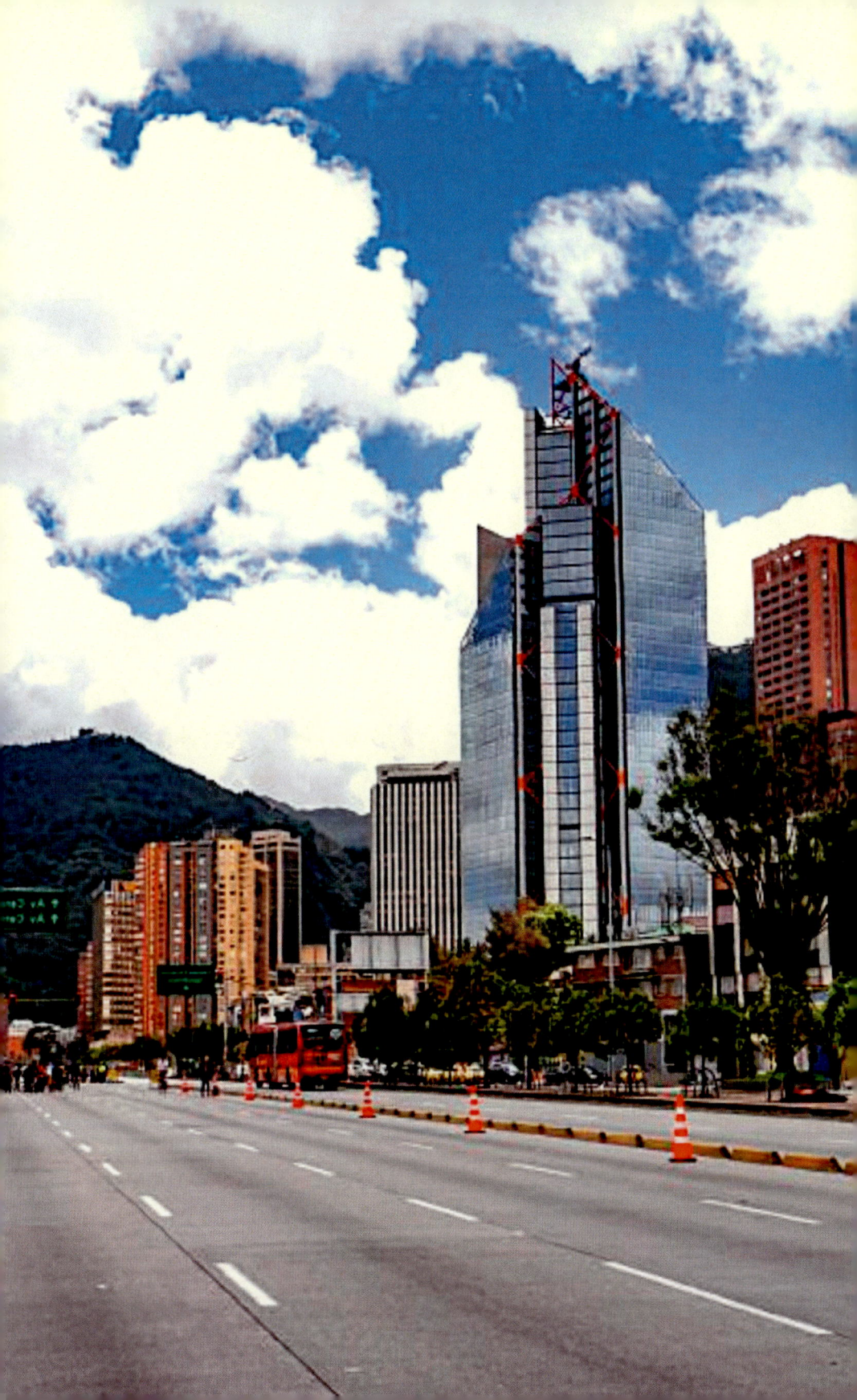

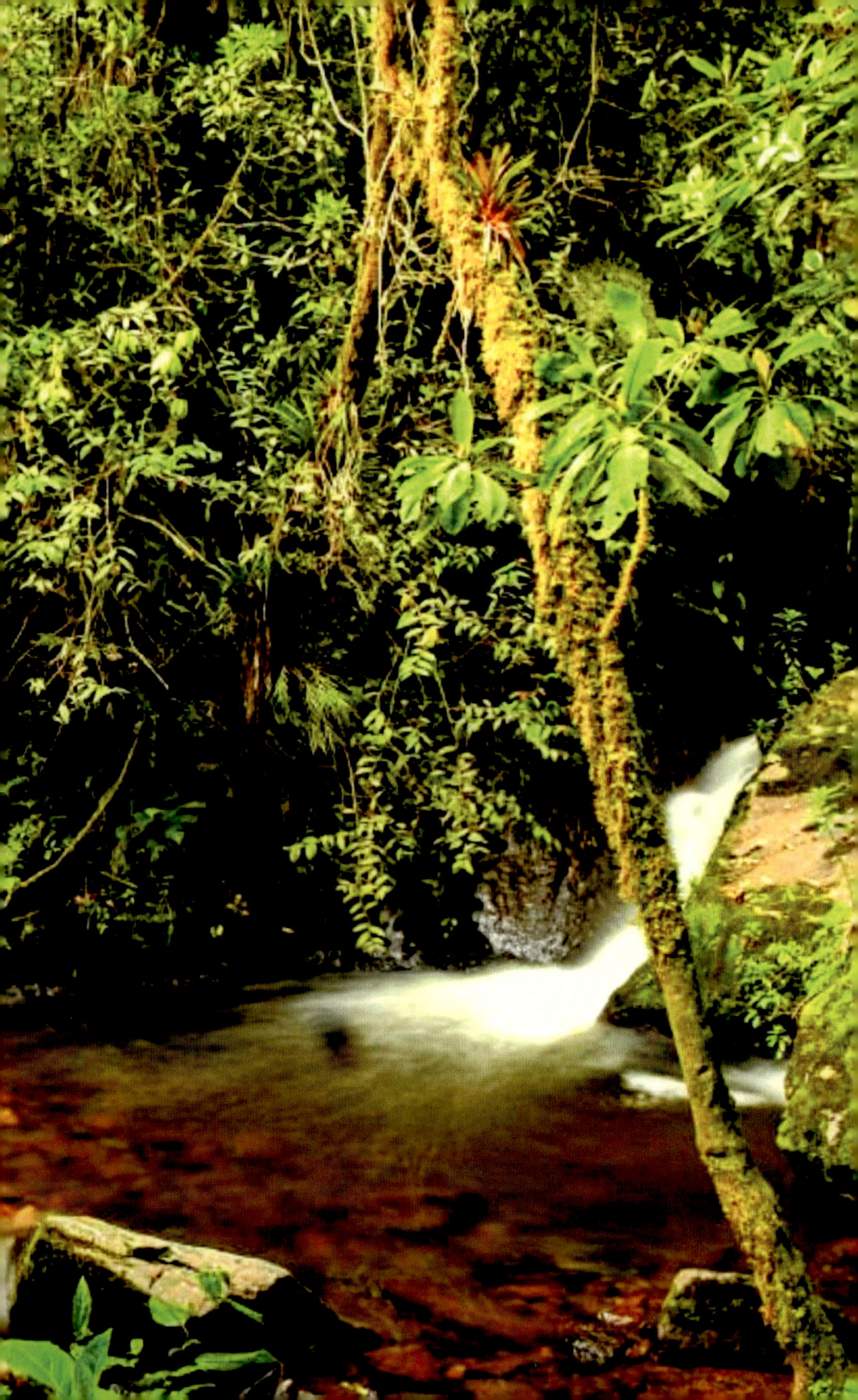

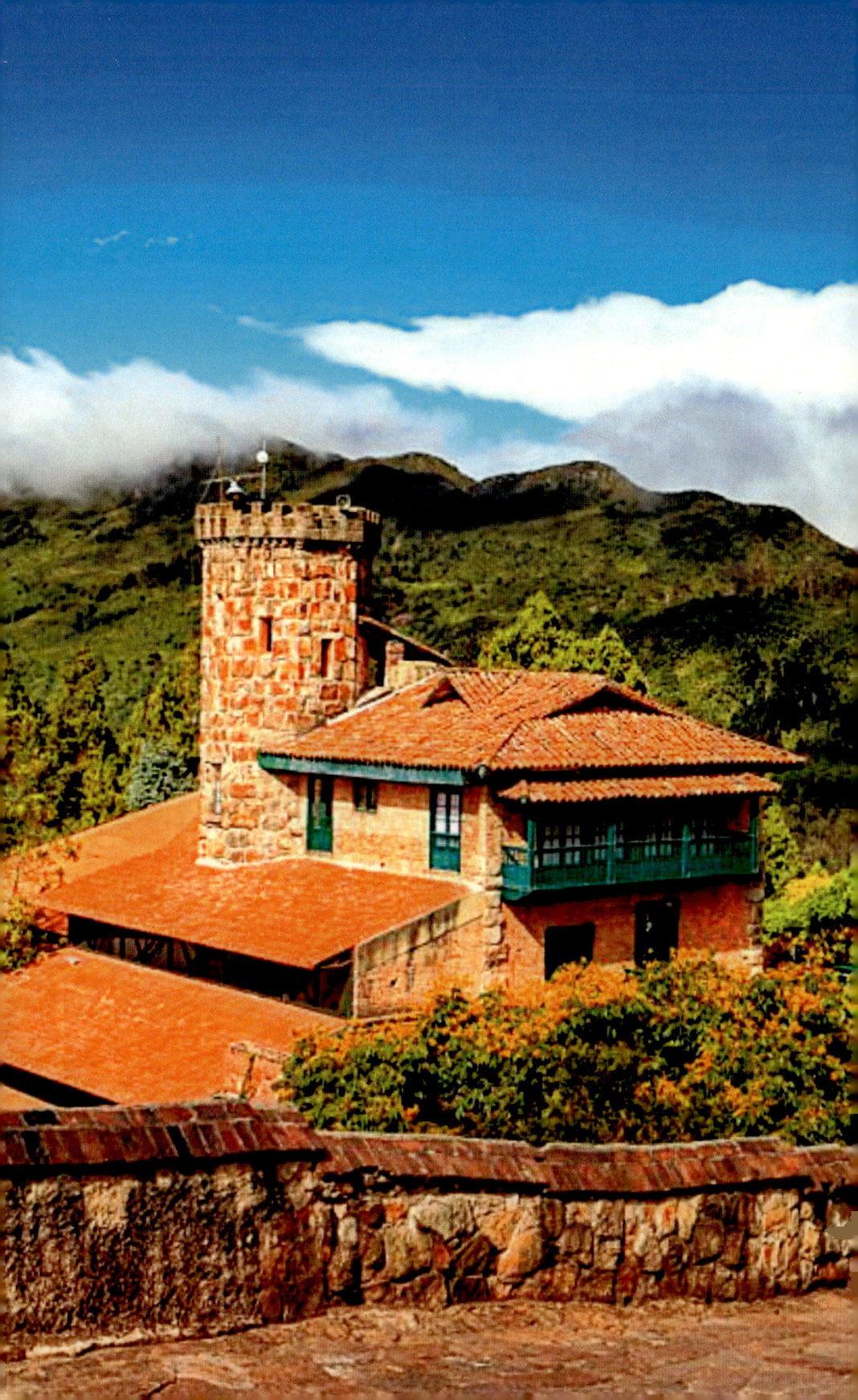

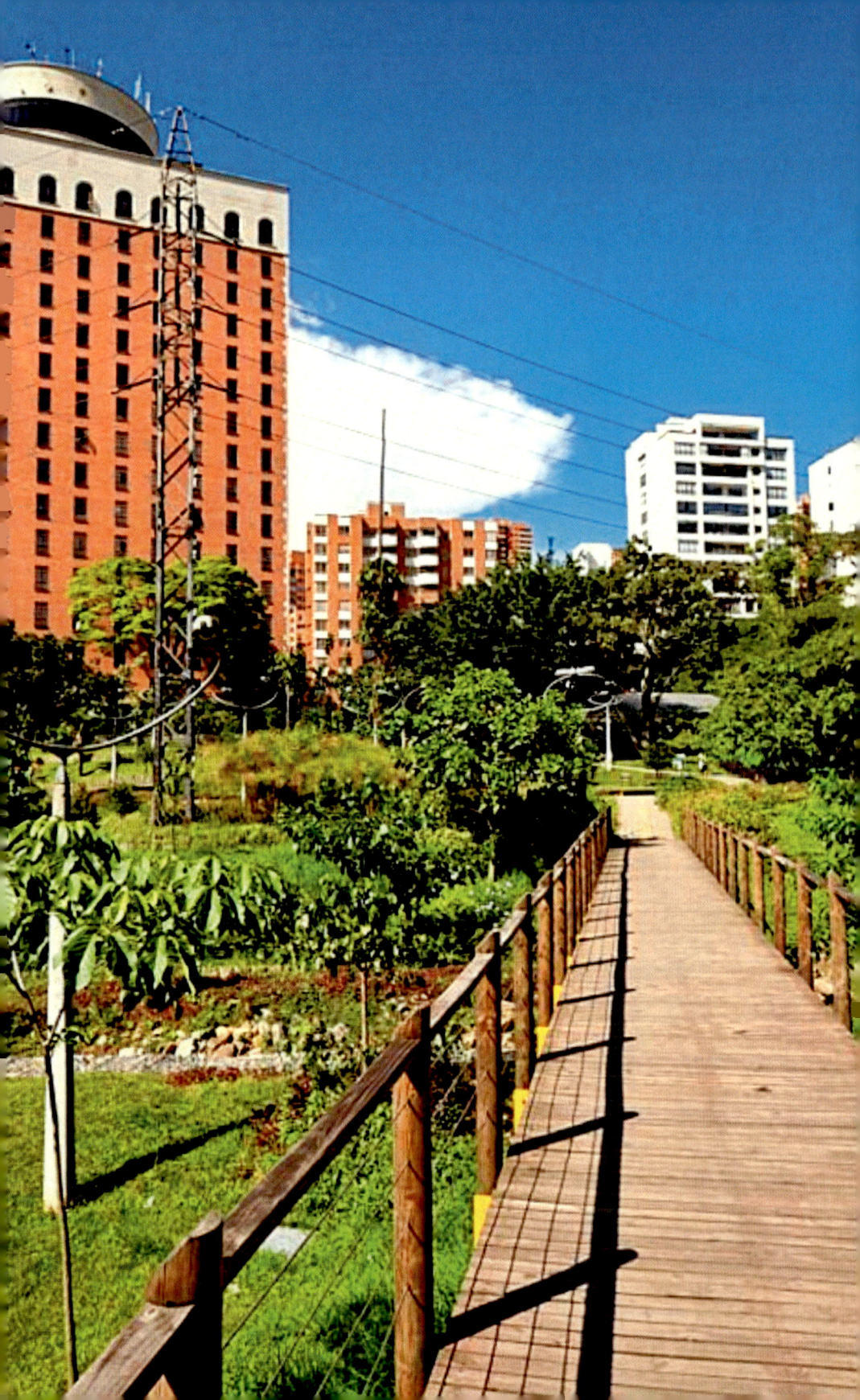

El Cove

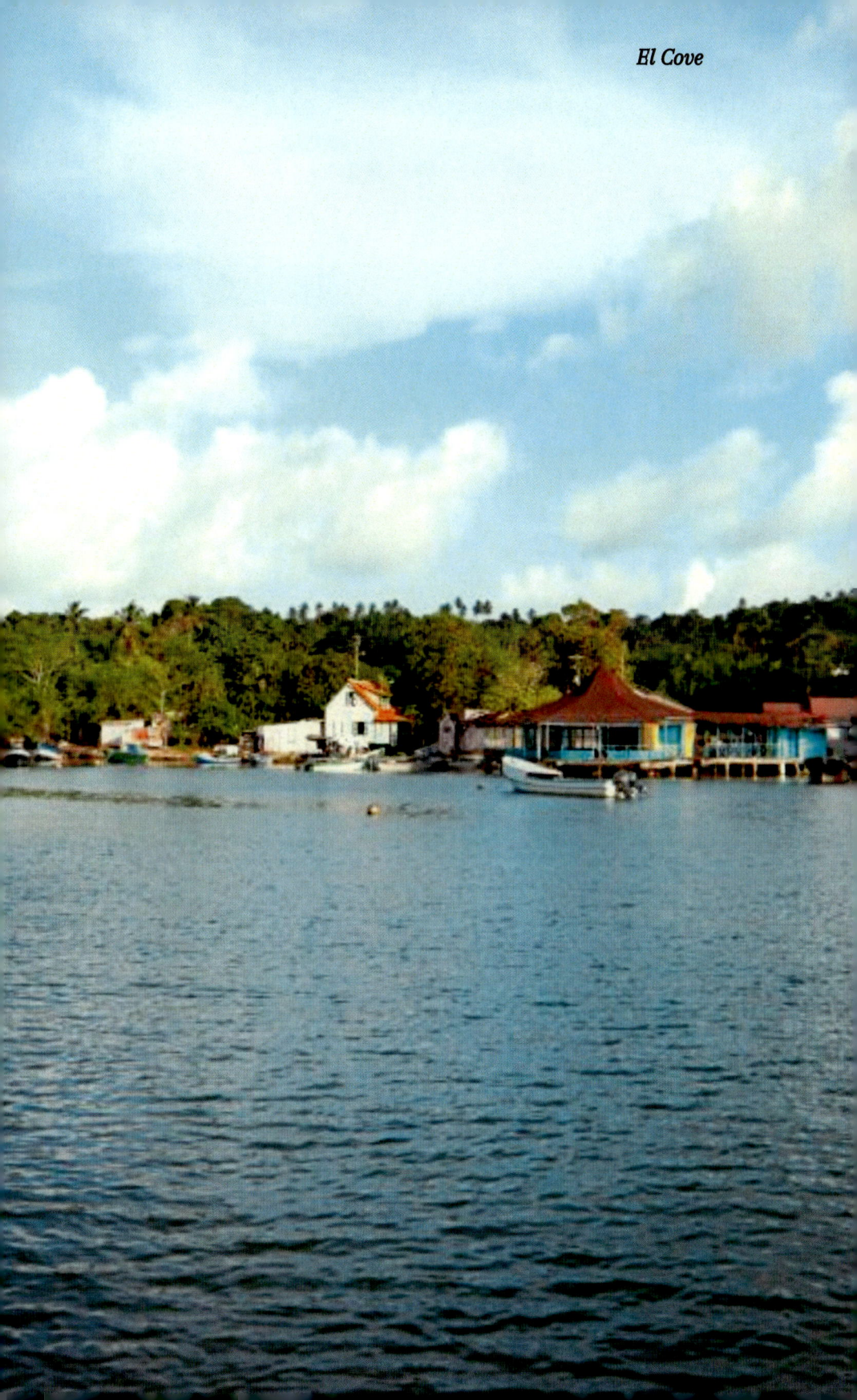

El Penon

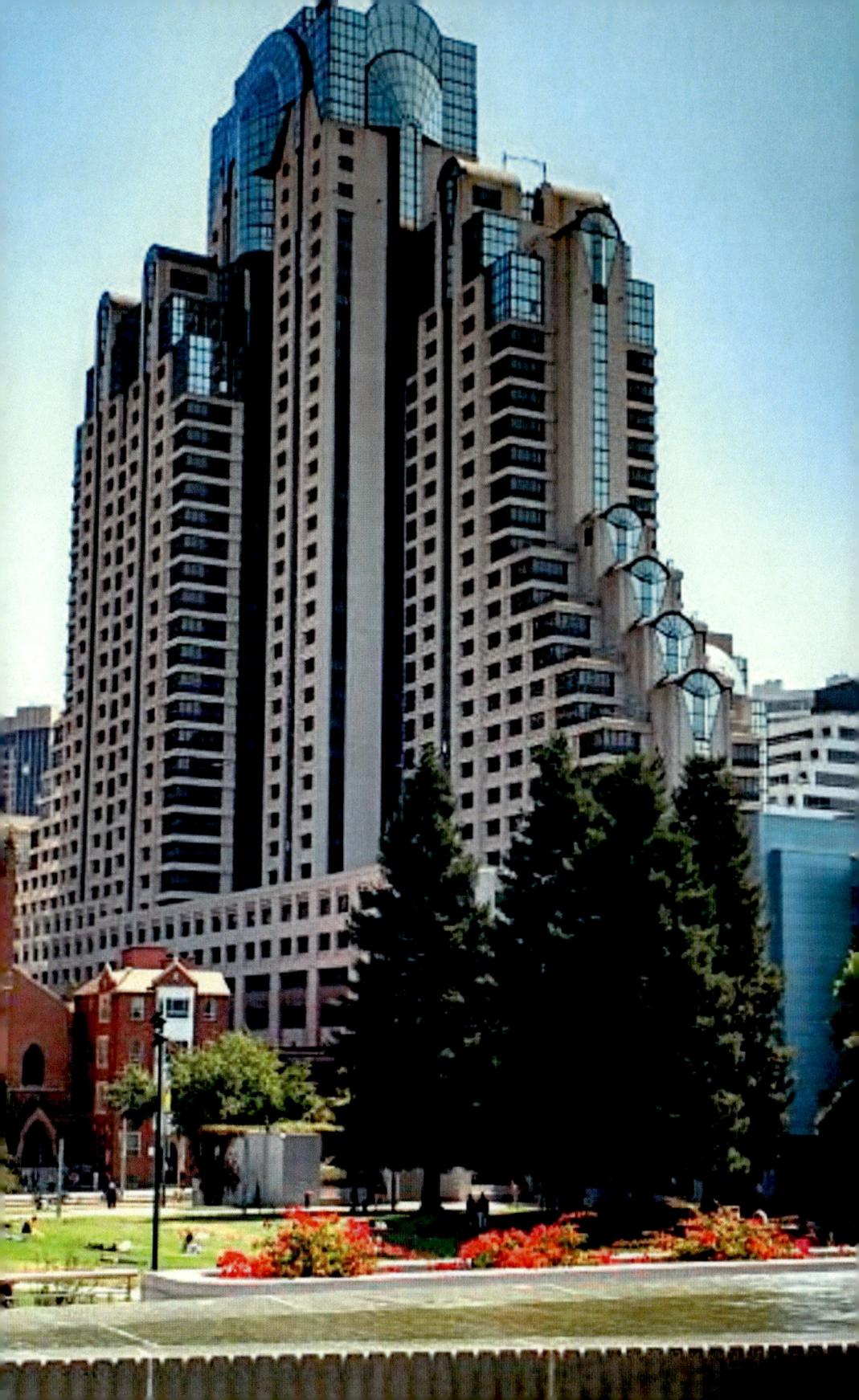

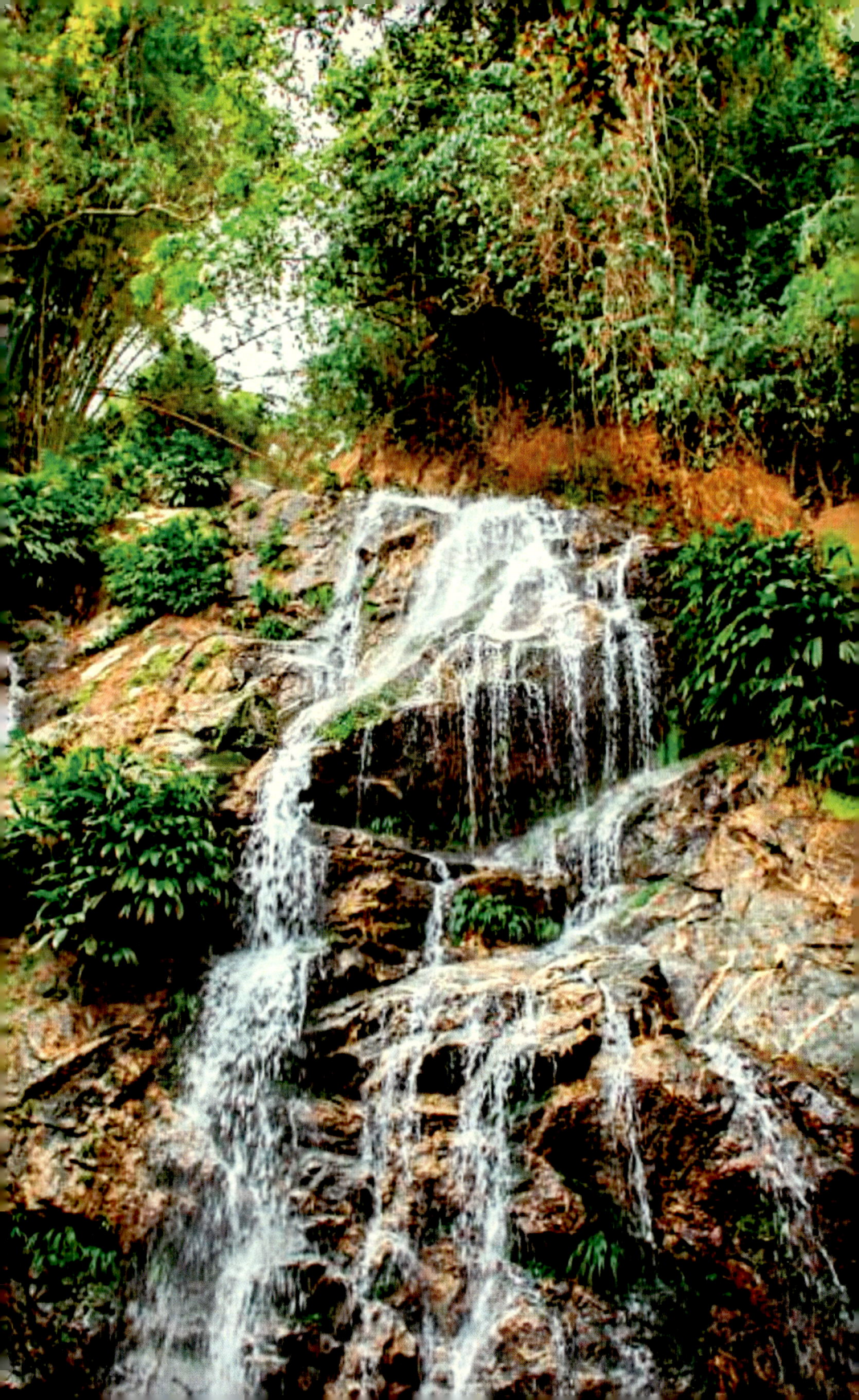

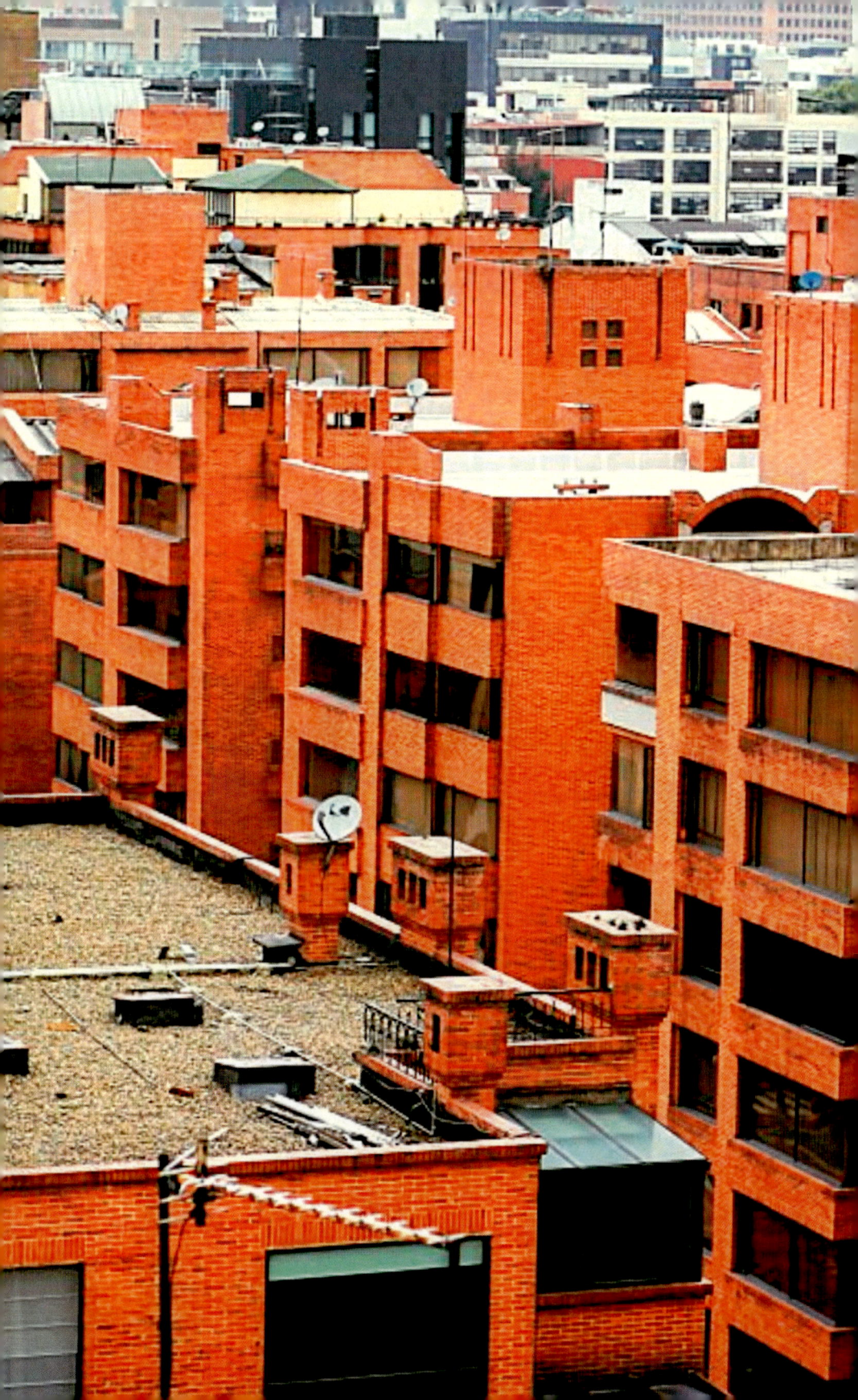

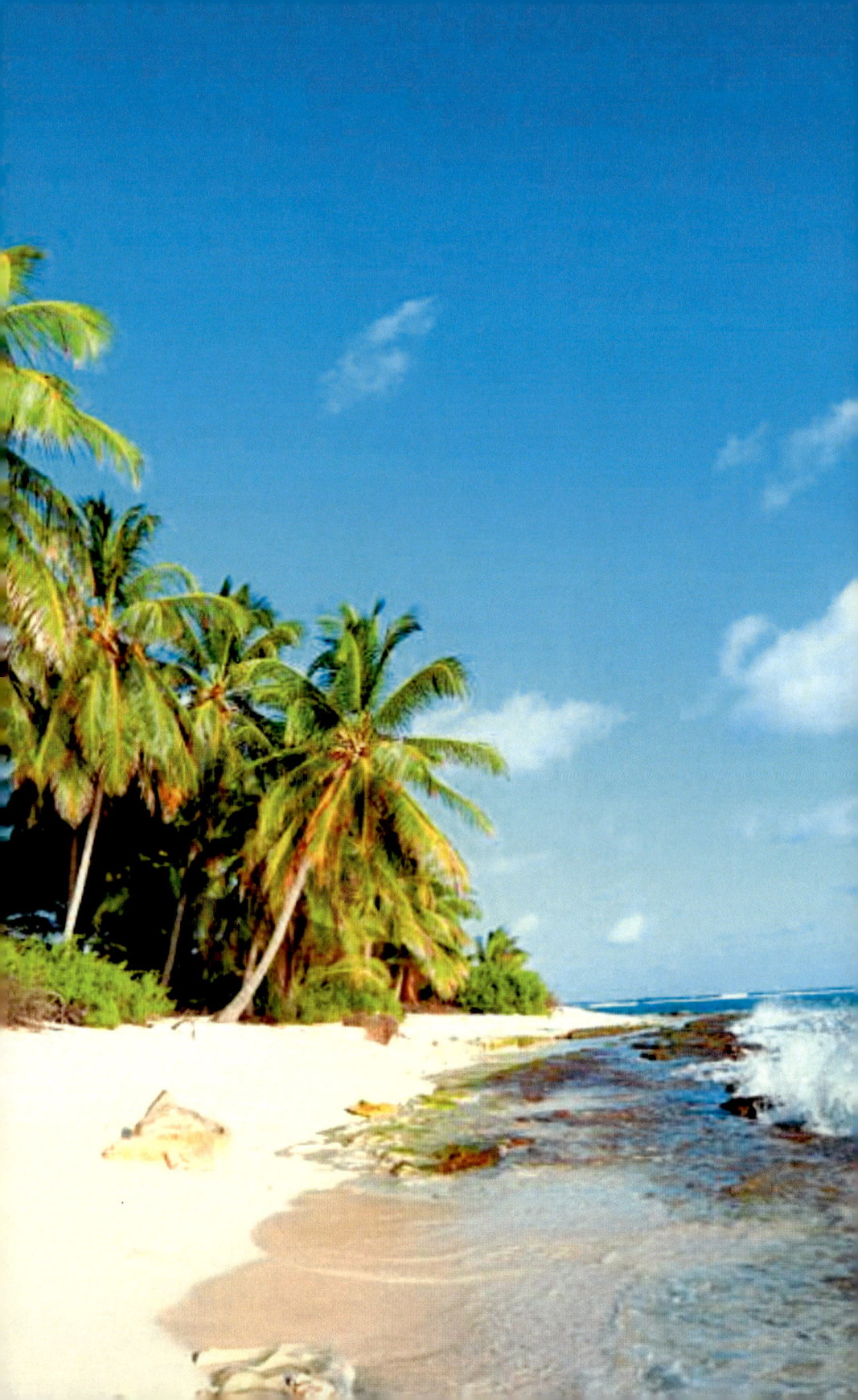

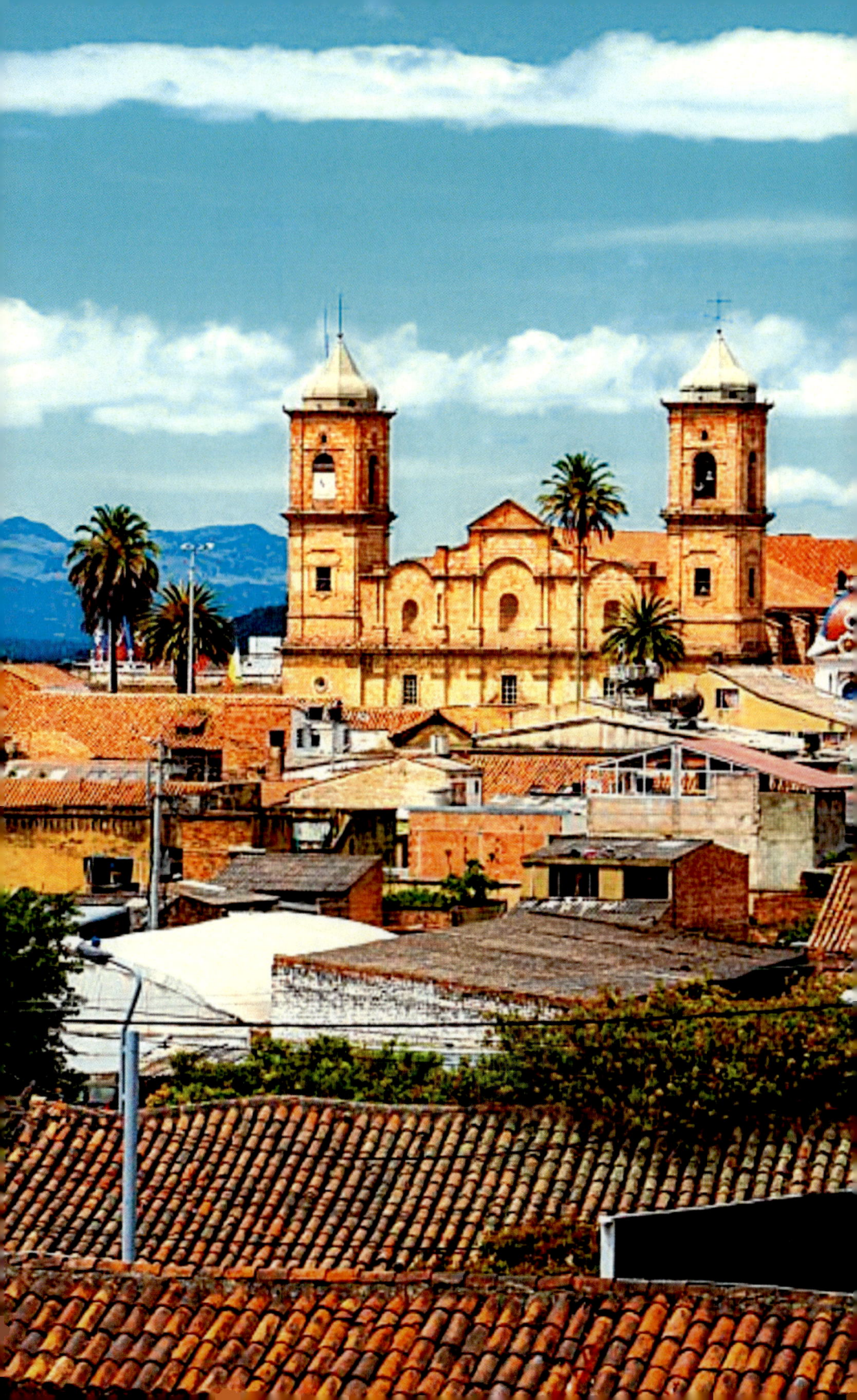

Chicamocha Canyon

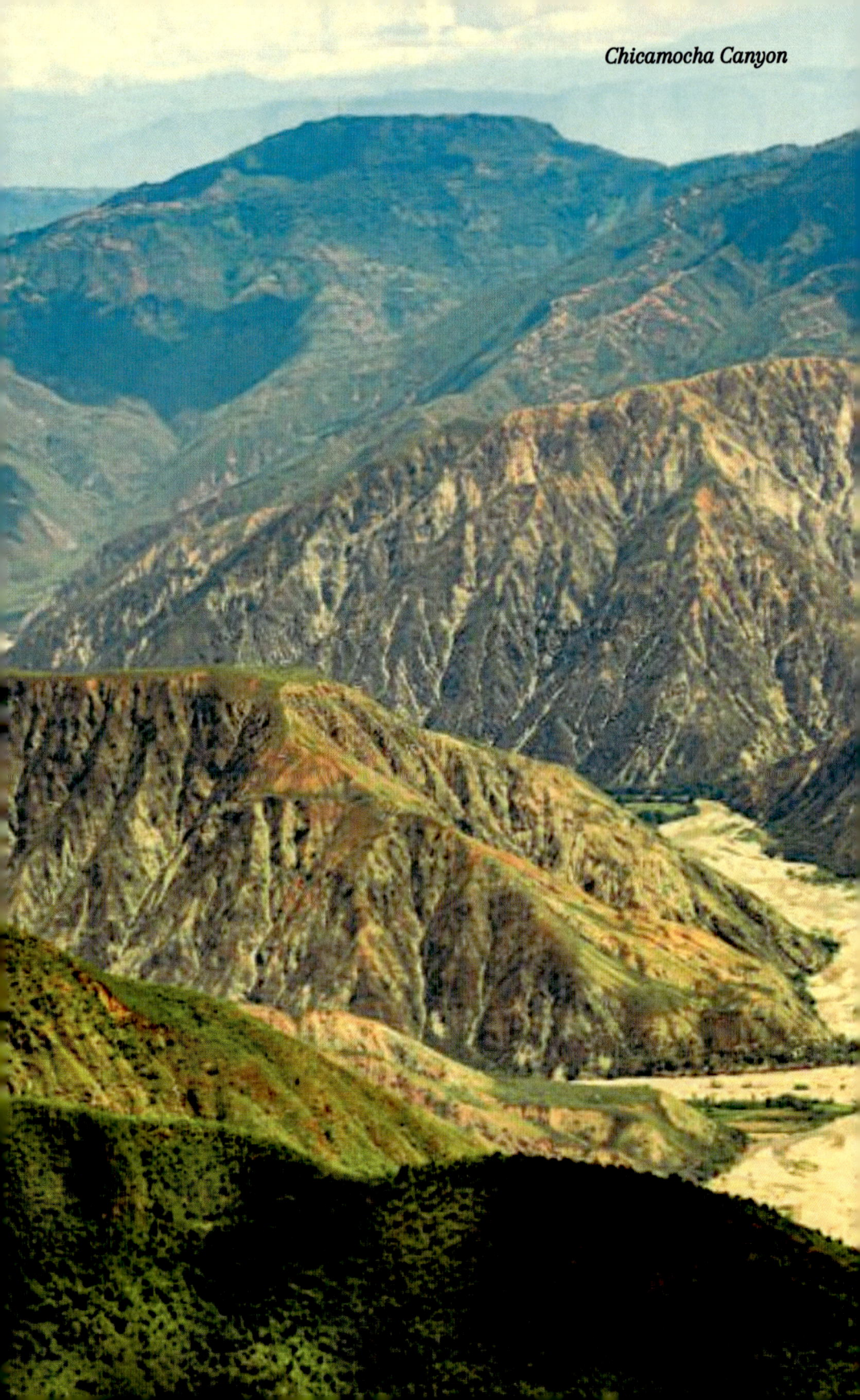

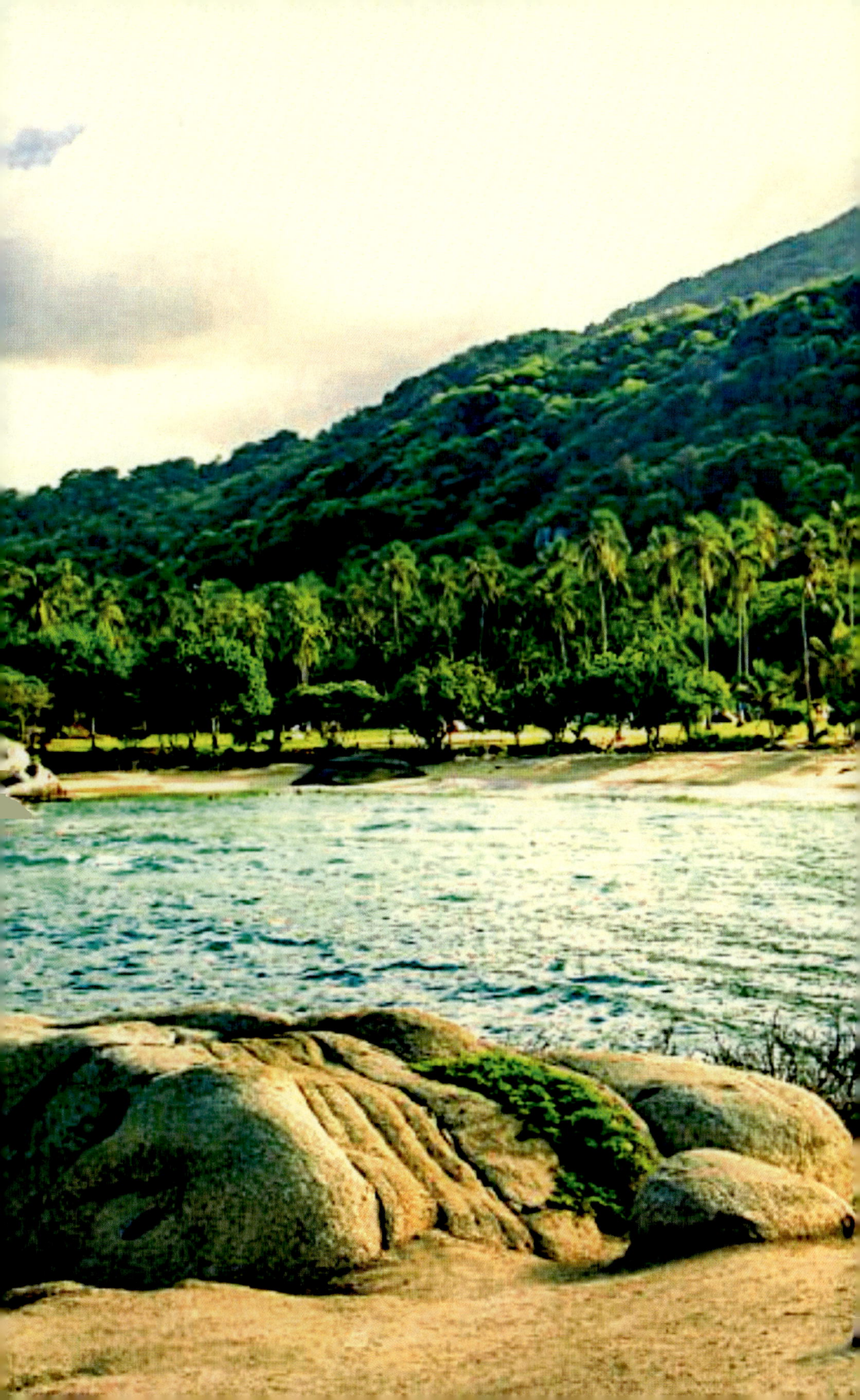

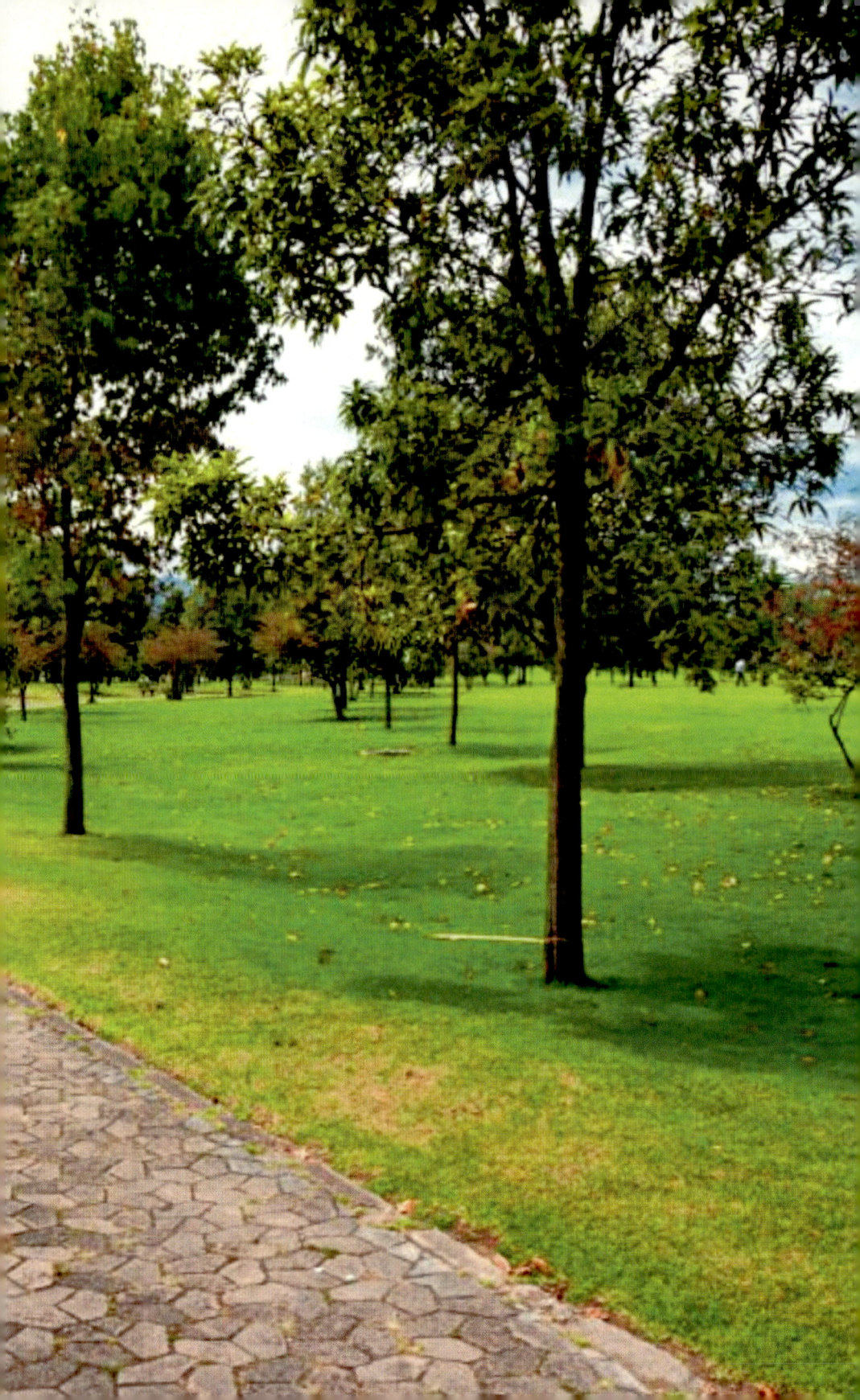

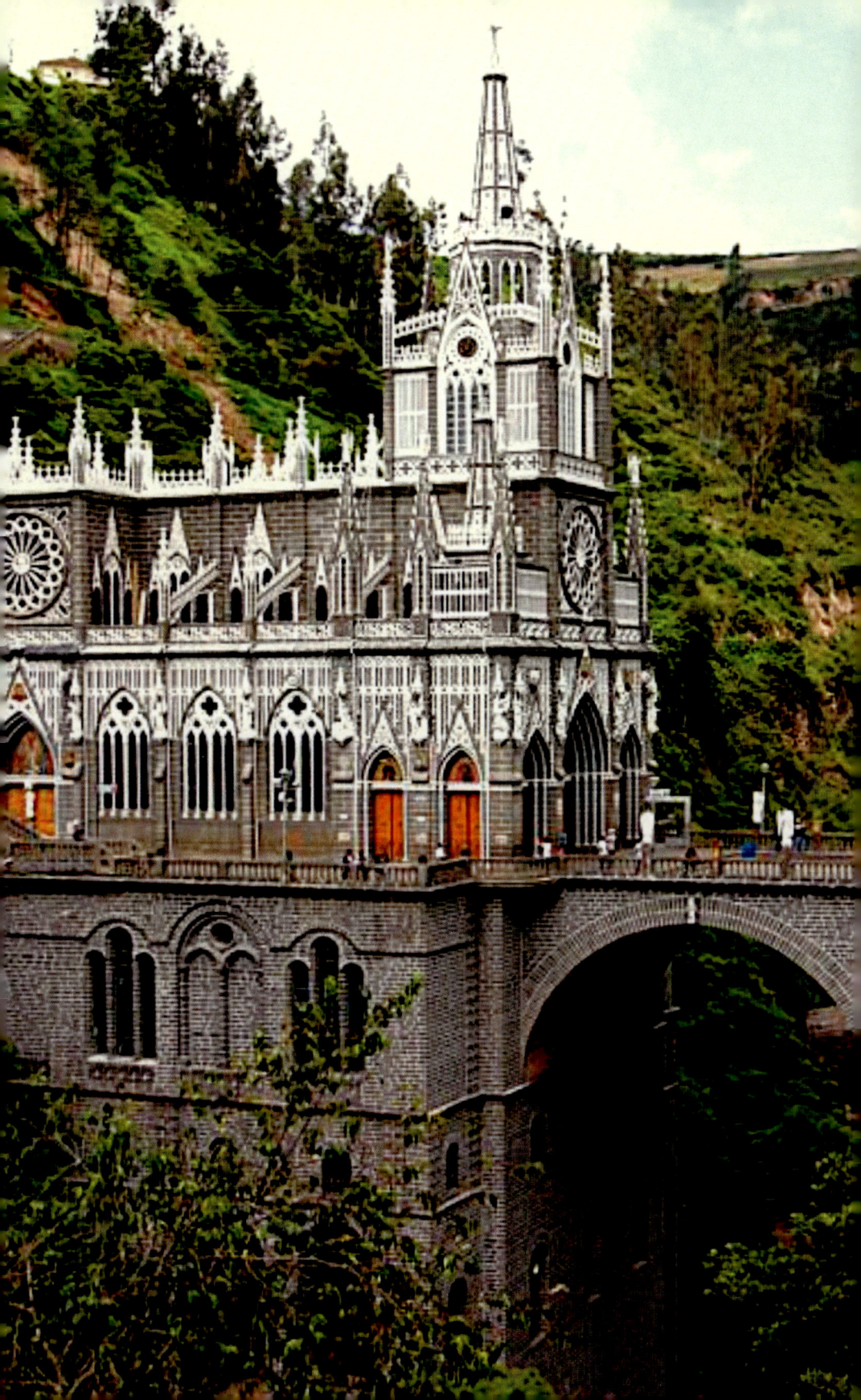

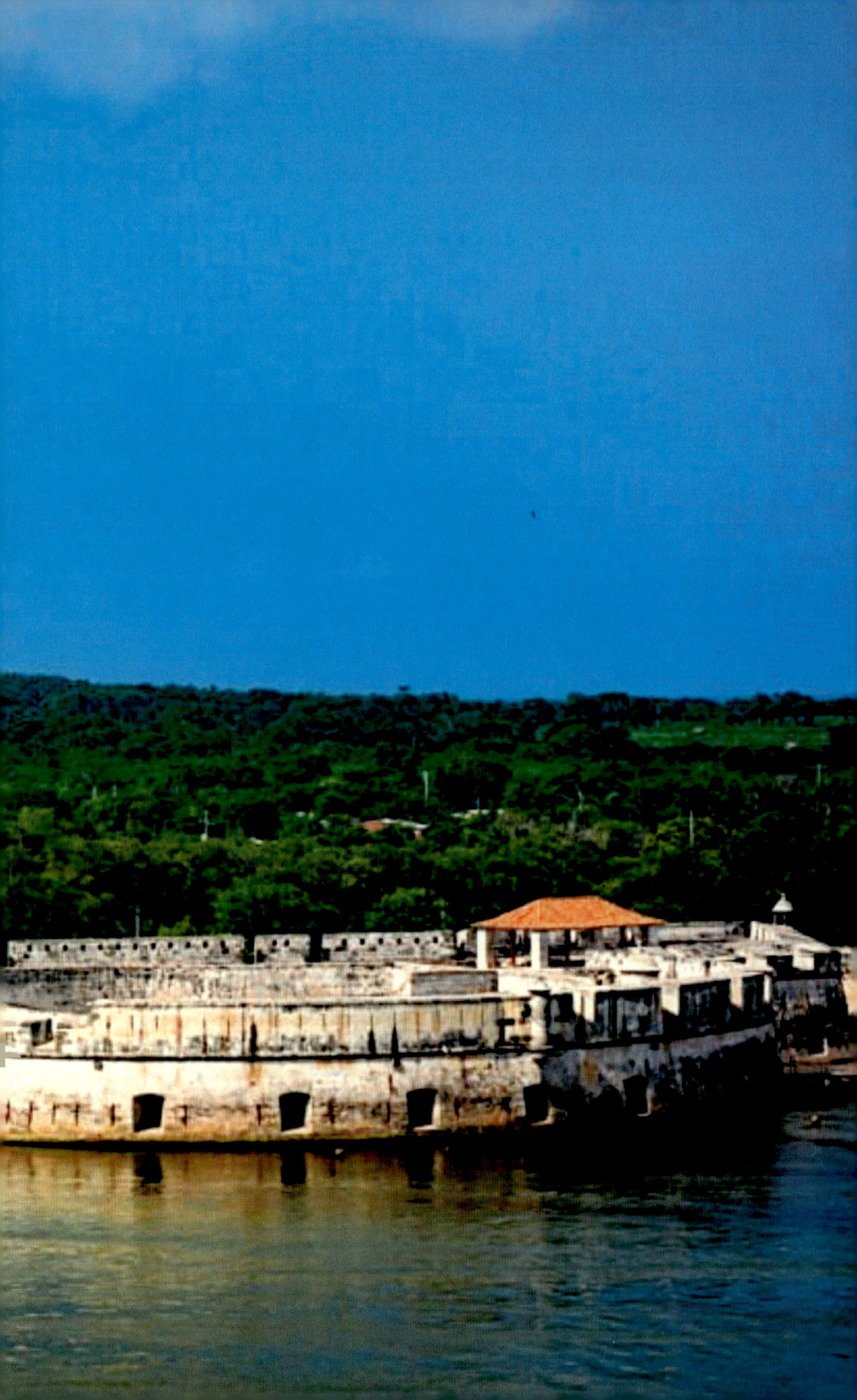

Castillo San Felipe de Barajas

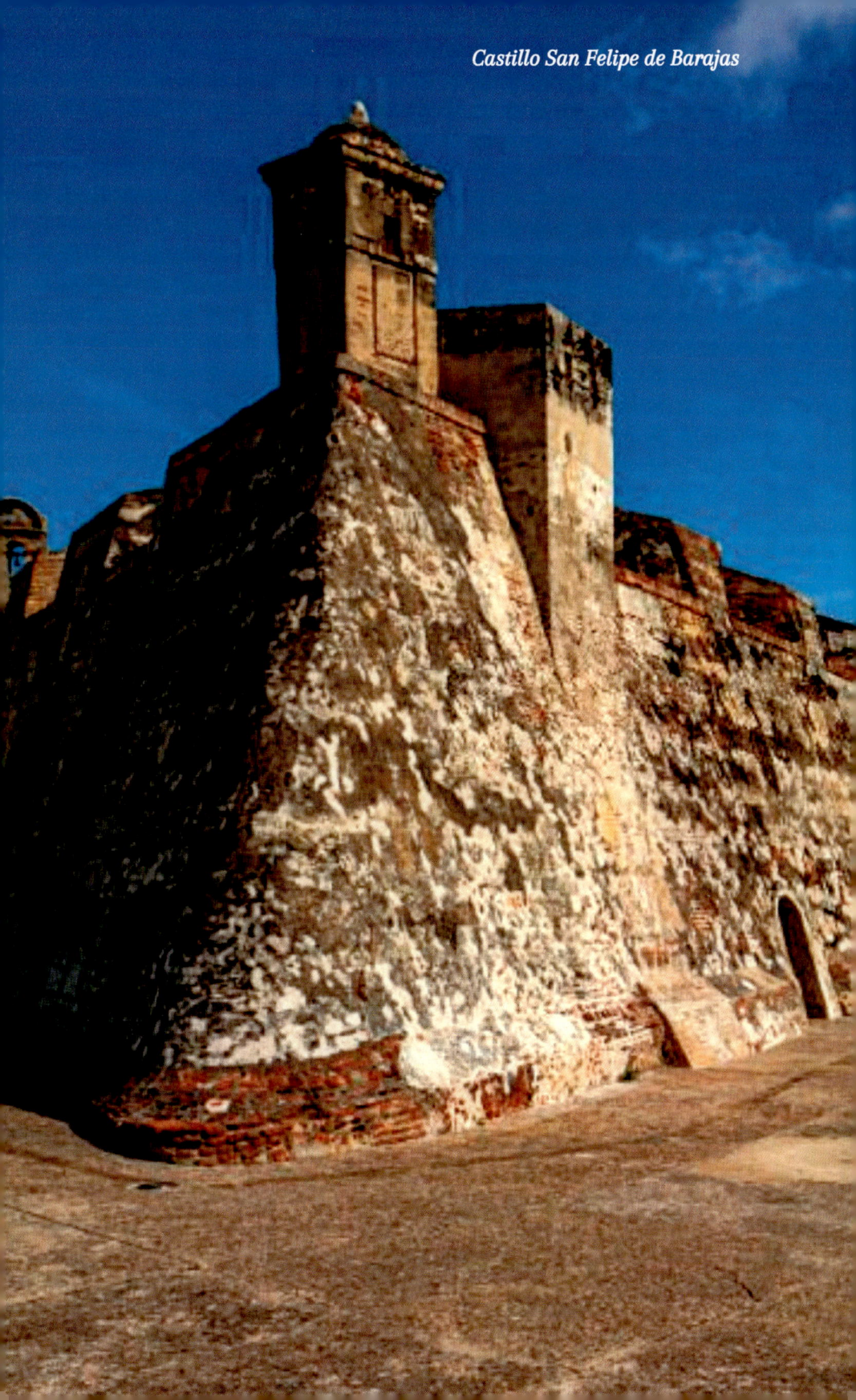

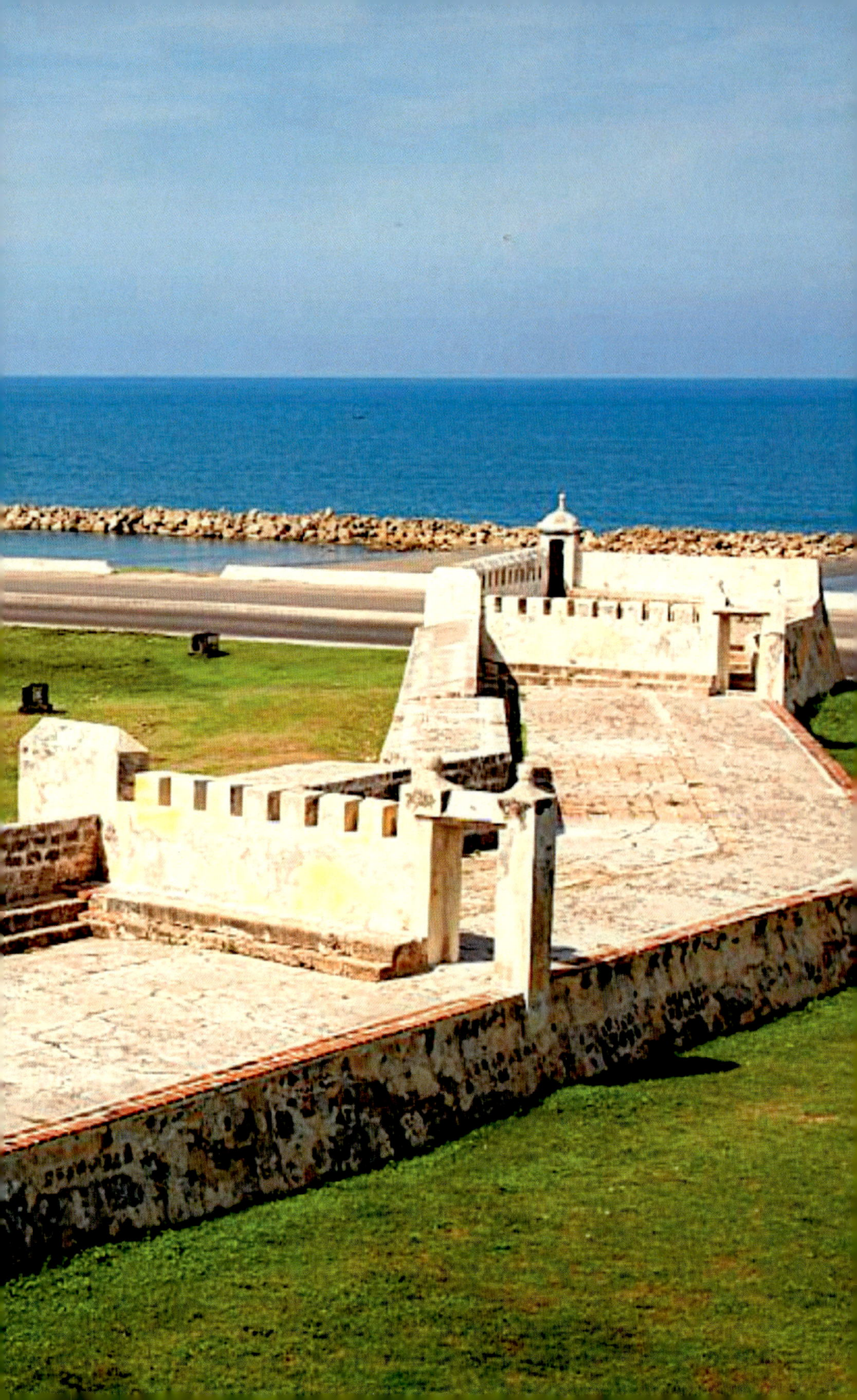

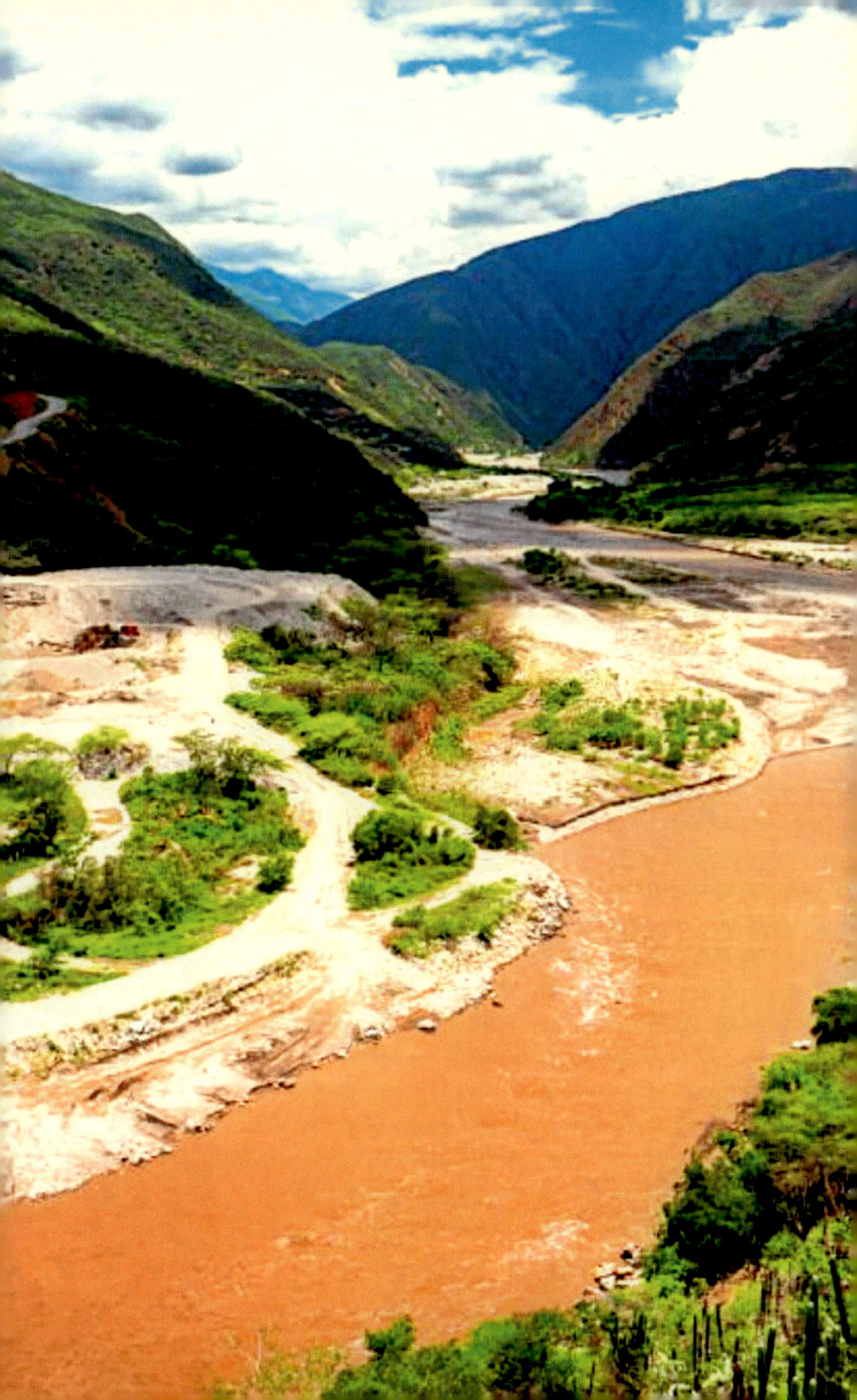

Ciudad Perdida

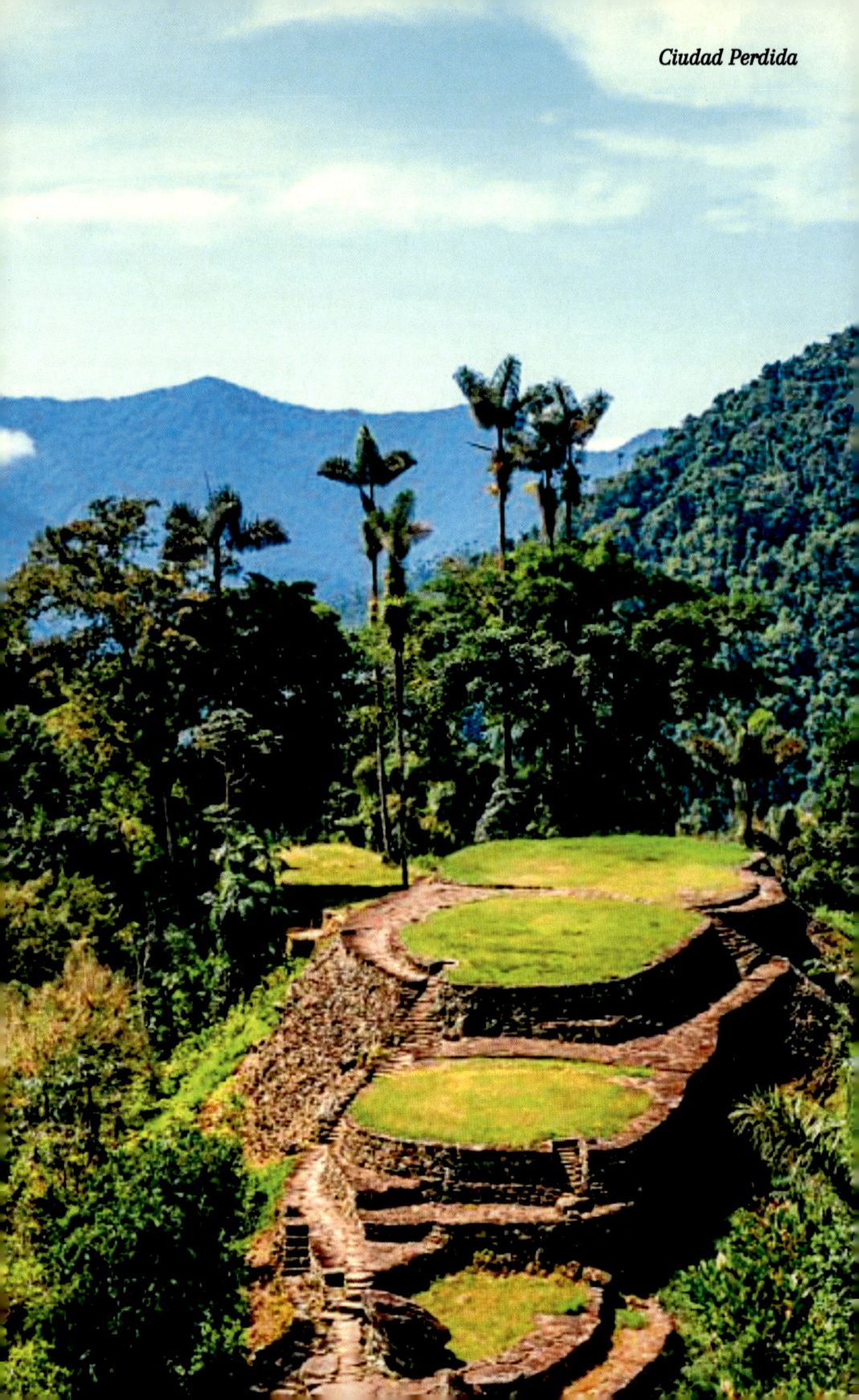

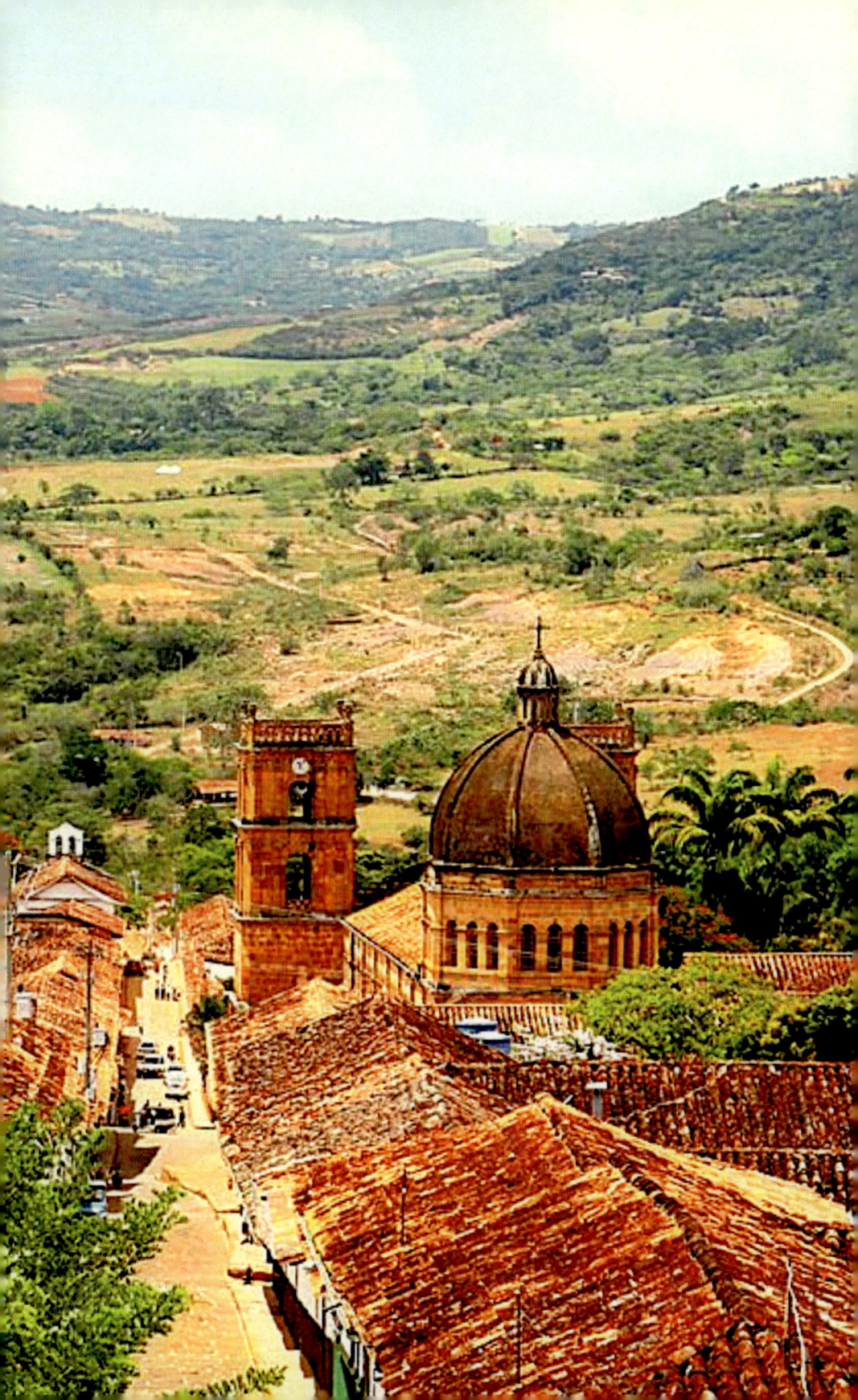

Made in United States
Orlando, FL
24 March 2025